Salon

Client Care

How to

Salon Client Care

How to

Maximize

Your Potential

for Success

J. Elaine Spear

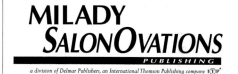

MILADY
SALONOVATIONS
PUBLISHING

a division of Delmar Publishers, an International Thomson Publishing company I(T)P*

3 Columbia Circle, P.O. Box 12519 • Albany, New York 12212-2519

Cover Design: J Squared Designs, Troy, NY

Milady Staff
Acquisitions Editor: Pamela Lappies
Project Editor: NancyJean Downey
Marketing Manager: Donna Lewis
Production and Art/Design Coordinator: Suzanne Nelson

COPYRIGHT © 1999
Milady Publishing
(a division of Delmar Publishers)
an International Thomson Publishing company
Printed in Canada
Distributed simultaneously in the United States of America and Canada

For more information, contact:
Milady/SalonOvations Publishing
3 Columbia Circle , Box 12519
Albany, New York 12212-2519

1 2 3 4 5 6 7 8 9 10 XXX 05 04 03 02 01 00 99

Library of Congress Cataloging-in-Publication Data

Spear, J. Elaine.
    Salon client care: how to maximize your potential for success / J. Elaine Spear.
      p.   cm.
    ISBN: 1-56253-349-5
    1. Beauty shops — Management.   I. Title.
TT965.S64   1998
646.7'2—dc21

98-19016
CIP

Dedication

This book is dedicated to my young

son, Robert Cody, who has taught

me that true success in life can

only be achieved through

balance. There is a

time for work,

play, and

love.

Table of Contents

Dedication   v
Preface   xi
About the Auuthor   xiii
Acknowledgments   xiv

Chapter 1   **Modernizing Your Approach**   1

    Creating Permanent Growth   1
    A Look at Salon History   2
    Caring for Today's Consumer 4
    The Customer Service Plan   7

Chapter 2   **Creating a Baseline for Care**   9

    Evaluating the State
     of Your Business   9
    Evaluating Your Salon Records 15
    Implementing the First Changes 21

Chapter 3   **Computerization**   23

    Gathering Information   23
    Software for Service   24
    Computerized Client
     Information   27
    Salon Analysis   31
    Creating a Complete Database 36
    Finding the Right System   40

Chapter 4	The Groundwork	41
	Perfecting Your Records	41
	Maintaining a Top-Notch Salon	45
	Client Surveys	47
	Funding Your Program	51
Chapter 5	Outlining a Plan	55
	Creating a Plan with Flexibility	55
	The Circle of Care	55
	By-products of Service	58
	A Sincere Welcome	59
	Pleasurable Care	63
	Prebooking	66
	A Tentative Outline	70
Chapter 6	Enactment of Change	75
	Conferring with Your Staff	75
	Staff Meetings	77
	8 Points of the Circle of Care	80
	Staff Surveys	94
Chapter 7	Creating a Contemporary Front Desk	97
	Redefining the Front Desk	97
	Organization of Training	97

Chapter 8	Rewarding Your Clientele	109
	System of Appreciation	109
	Goodwill Gifting Programs	113
	New Client Incentives	117
	Seasonal Gift Packs	122
	Embracing the Programs	123
Chapter 9	Acts of Pleasure	125
	More than Pampering	125
	Acts of Wellness	125
	Finishing Touches	130
Chapter 10	The Art of Retrieval	131
	Second Chances at Success	131
	The Retrieval Process	132
	Achieving Retention	136
	Index	139

Preface

When Milady Publishing first accepted my offer to write a book about contemporary client care, I was absolutely thrilled. My salon ownership days were freshly behind me and I felt that I wanted to pass on my success to others. But while working on this book, I discovered something far more valuable than anything I could share myself.

As salon owners, we are incredibly isolated from our peers. When I launched my second career as a journalist for our industry, I began receiving volumes of quality business information from high-powered salon owners throughout the world. And while their information continues to be rich with diversity, it has always contained a common theme: salon systems. Over the long haul, salons that are successful implement systems in their businesses to ensure a consistent result. If you want payroll done every week by 11:00, you set up a system. To ensure technical excellence, you need an educational system. And, if you want your clients to receive an extremely positive visit every time they come to your salon, you need a system of care.

Salon Client Care shares how all salons can offer exquisite care to their clients. Perfecting this system not only promotes a steady increase in the number of clients you serve, but also in your salon personnel. In a business that can appear and disappear in the blink of an eye, this is indeed an important strategy to embrace. And, because all salons have different needs and temperaments, *Salon Client Care* also allows salon owners to customize their own programs to perfectly match their individual situations.

MY STORY

When I first began in the beauty business, I worked as a stylist in a quiet area of Southern California. The salon owner was extremely nice although she was not very tuned into her business. Working there became increasingly difficult because we lacked a client care system, as well as nearly all details required to keep a business running smoothly. I remember how frustrating it was to have no-shows on my books, spend precious minutes hunting for clean smocks for clients, and wading through piles of hair left behind by others because cleanliness was an individual decision and not the policy of the salon. We were often slow, then busy, then slow again and no one could ever figure out why except to say that things were slow everywhere. Slow business was blamed on the road work, the weather, or the economy. We did not confirm our appointments, kept a few client cards on a first-name basis, and did not miss people for years after they quit coming to our salon.

One day near Christmas, I was working on one client while another was sitting in the shampoo area waiting for her tint to process. My color client, approached me and asked for tissue. I searched everywhere, but found none. The owner did not put a lot of energy into taking care of the small things that made our clients' visits more enjoyable. Ten minutes later, and starting to panic, I turned to the receptionist and asked her to please get a tissue for my client who by that time had a serious problem. I returned to the client in my chair and did not notice until a few minutes later that my color client was sitting in the shampoo area with a big roll of pink toilet paper on her lap, tissue strung up to her nose. Horrified, I turned to the receptionist who shrugged and said, "Hey, it works. We haven't had Kleenex in three weeks." I went immediately to my client and she told me in no uncertain terms, "It is either me or this salon." I could not have agreed more and put in my notice of resignation that day.

THE PURSUIT OF QUALITY

Since that incident, quality care has become my lifelong pursuit. Eventually I found a professional salon that offered me a great education in client care as well as technical instruction. My own systems have sprouted from these early teachings. I learned that good care required more than a quality service and good stock. It also encompassed every experience clients have with their salon. Today, the importance of exquisite care is even greater. With our clientele growing ever more sophisticated in the ways of service as well as beauty, salons need to balance great services with even better overall care. This not only means making what we already do better, but also adopting new habits that will improve service.

The contemporary client care program encourages salon owners to dedicate themselves to creating an accurate database that will reward as well as track their clientele, and to make all the small details of their salon important parts of their overall business. It involves decisions by staff members, as well as salon owners, and helps set up systems that enable salons to run efficiently at all times. *Salon Client Care* also encourages pleasurable acts such as chair massage and aromatherapy as part of routine salon services, and doing such meaningful things as systematically prebooking all clients, to increase gross earnings by as much as 50 percent! What advertising campaign can promise this?

CREATING A STABLE, VIABLE BUSINESS

As a previous salon owner, I know that even when embracing a quality client care system, owning a salon can often be both heaven and hell. We gain and lose clients and staff for a variety of reasons that often defy logic. But, with a successful client care system, these highs and lows become cleansing acts rather than disasters. If you lose clients because they have never been satisfied, a great client care system will not help retain them. Nor will it retain staff members who are anxious to embark on new careers. But, it will keep those who are meaningful to your operation, and dramatically reduce defections by stylists who, without a good care system, will drift to other salons because of frustration and failure. Maintaining the cutting edge of care, as well as style, is a people-pleasing balance that will keep your chairs full and your staff in complete harmony with your salon. Enjoy!

About the Author

A stylist/salon owner since 1977, Spear is now a full-time beauty and wellness writer for numerous publications including *Self, Salon News, DaySpa* and *Professional Cosmetics*. When she retired from the salon business in 1993, her salon was realizing over $1,000,000 in annual sales. With her exceptional education and promotional background, Spear specializes in business, beauty, and wellness information for beauty professionals and consumers. She is also expert in developing and promoting beauty businesses on the Internet.

Acknowledgments

I would like to thank all the wonderful people who have taken time out of their own lives to create, gather, and donate material for our *Salon Client Care* book.

Many thanks to Kelly Taggert, co-owner of Purely Visual in Tustin, California, for her generous photography for this book. And to her partner, David Winterhalter, for photographing me "just right."

Also, thanks to Salon Transcripts of Woodland Hills, California, for donating their time and expertise in creating all of our sample computer reports. The resources needed to accomplish this act of generosity are gratefully acknowledged!

And to all the salons who openly shared information for all our readers, thank you! Meeting such wonderful salon owners and staffs has been both a delightful and enlightening experience. They are proof that the more knowledge you acquire, the more open you are to sharing it with others!

The Publisher would like to thank the following professionals for their expertise in reviewing this book: Patti Ferraro, Boca Raton, FL; Florence Hogan, Sterling Heights, MI; Sharon MacGregor, Bloomingburg, NY; and Lois Wiskur, Pierre, SD.

chapter 1

Modernizing Your Approach

1. Creating permanent growth
2. The cost of doing business
3. A look at salon history
4. Defining contemporary client care
5. Customizing for success

HOTopic

CREATING PERMANENT GROWTH

Owning a salon is often like riding a world-class roller coaster. Filled with dramatic highs and death-defying lows, it is a thrilling experience that leaves many salon owners clinging to their seats and praying for level ground.

On the front lines of the beauty business, complete success is often elusive. It waits for us just around the bend, creating intermittent feelings of victory and defeat. We often build up one part of our business only to lose ground in another. And, despite sincere efforts, the majority of working artists have many busy days but never fully-built careers.

The constant replenishment of clients and staff experienced by most salons not only exhausts bank accounts, but also the very core of our creative spirit. And, if you believe your business is the exception, take a moment to check your records. How many stylists have left you since you opened your business? How many clients in your salon records have not returned in the last 90 days? The last year? The last five years?

The Cost of Doing Business

If you provide each one of your stylists only one new client per week, during the course of two years every artist on your staff will receive at least 100 new clients compliments of your salon. In today's economy, it takes approximately $45.00 to attract a new client. This figure is based on advertising and general overhead. So, if your salon has eight chairs, in two year's time you have invested $36,000:

    8 x 100 new clients = 800 clients
    800 clients x $45.00 = $36,000.00

If your retention level is 50 percent or less, your loss on this investment could be $18,000 or more.

Stylists who never become completely built will always need a steady supply of new clients. The next time your bank account is empty, look here first!

Exquisite Client Care

You will always have a percentage of clients and staff who come and go, but the majority of people are truly looking for a great place to remain and be happy. Let that business be yours! In order to have that dynamic draw, though, you will need a plan: One that ensures that all clients consistently receive exquisite care each time they visit your salon. In doing so, you will be joining a new chapter in the history of our business. Customer service defined as "a great smile and a good style" is dead. Today, clients want an extraordinary experience in exchange for their loyalty.

A LOOK AT SALON HISTORY

In the 1930s, hair salons thrived while other businesses failed. It was the Great Depression. During that time, people could not buy hair dye over the counter and perms were definitely in the hands of professionals only. If you wanted to look your best, you had to go to the beauty salon. How nice!

The majority of married women did not work outside the home and beauty salons provided a feminine meeting place where they could catch up on local news, relax, and briefly be cared for by others. To be a successful salon during this period, the shop needed to be friendly, conveniently located, and offer styles that could last an entire week.

In 1940, the hairdressing industry was given both a blessing and a blow when the cold wave arrived on the beauty scene. Not long after, over-the-counter manufacturers began retailing cold waves to consumers. Permanent hair dye, formerly the domain of beauty salons only, also became an over-the-counter commodity. For the first time, women could perm and color their hair at home. And, despite the inferior products available over-the-counter, our industry began to significantly feel the economic results. Unequipped to handle these turns of events, salons were helpless to even slow the defection process. Marketing and sophisticated client care remained things for future generations to sort out.

In the 1930s, hair salons thrived while other businesses failed.

In the late 1950s, fashion introduced the fated beehive. And, as it blossomed and turned into Grecian, dancing petal curls and more, the beauty industry experienced a much needed resurgence of salon clients. A simple French twist became a swirling vortex of unimaginable complexity. Hair was bleached to ultra-pale shades, toned with the most delicate of pastels, and pasted absolutely stiff with hair lacquer. Women, proving that they were still slaves to fashion, not only returned to the salon in droves, but snuggled up next to their husbands at night with their hair wrapped in toilet paper, keeping their 'dos in place for days.

For the hairdressers who excelled in teasing (some even sharpened their combs), as well as styles that would have remained immortalized if it were not for hot water (you had to melt the lacquer first!), it meant that business was good. And, during this time, the same principles of client care that were used so diligently in the 1930s were still practiced without any thoughts of changing. The true inadequacies of client care only emerged when the weekly client faded from view. Even then, it was not acknowledged until decades later.

We embraced the idea of being professionals rather than tradespeople.

The Hairdressing Revolution

During our entire hairdressing history prior to the introduction of the precision cut, haircuts were very cheap. Good color, an average haircut, and a great set were what women really needed. It was not a terribly lucrative career, nor did it offer retirement or health benefits. But it was a stable paycheck and a predictable routine. Then came the revolution. It hit our shores abruptly and shook every pillar and beam of our industry with such fierceness that not only was our approach redefined, but also our heroes and our methods of doing business. It was the mid-1960s and the blow-dryer had arrived on the scene. Elaborate hairdos fell by the wayside and with them, our entire industry as we knew it disintegrated seemingly overnight.

The new styling wave began in London, led by such hairdressing legends as Vidal Sassoon and Paul Mitchell. They pioneered precision cutting and blow drying in America with such charisma and talent that stylists everywhere embraced their methods with passion and relief. Our field opened up for thousands of new budding stylists who eagerly joined our changing world dreaming of becoming celebrities themselves.

Our leaders taught us a new way to walk, talk, and look at ourselves. We became styling salons, servicing both men and women. Our techniques and overwhelming resurgence nearly made the barber industry extinct. We embraced the idea of being professionals rather than tradespeople. And, shedding the old image of long hours with low pay, the new breed of hairdressers flocked to training classes that taught the new artistry of "haircutting," and demanded higher prices for salon services.

Yet, despite the excitement of these times, earnings plummeted. Stylists who previously only needed 50 clients to be fully booked, were suddenly faced with the enormity of finding 300 eager souls to exclusively use their services. The intimate client/hairdresser ties were broken as our clients' appointments stretched to six weeks or more. Keeping existing clients as well as finding new clients became both a puzzle and a challenge.

The New Age of Client Care

Hair salons and hairdressers were gaining technical skills but losing in most other areas. Client care and marketing were foreign words to stylists, and salon owners had no education to make up the gap. It began taking years instead of months to build clientele. Many salons could not keep up. Suddenly clients could choose between dozens of stylists eager for their business. No longer obligated by the weekly visit ritual and the relationship it entailed, they began to "shop around," change, and move with amazing frequency. Despite this glaring reality, it was not until years later that our industry discovered that the need to create great client handling skills was just as important as maintaining high technical expertise. By this time, many good stylists were averaging poverty level wages and the expected stay in the industry was less than five years.

Thirty-five years after the hairdressing revolution, with many mistakes and triumphs experienced along the way, our industry has now evolved into one that promotes success at many levels. Good stylists may not always be busy and good client-care staff may not be booked completely. But good stylists who are also client-care specialists are thriving and will continue to do so well into the 21st century. It is yet another new beginning for our industry.

CARING FOR TODAY'S CONSUMER

Just as our industry has evolved, so have the tastes of the people we serve. The consumer of the late 1990s is distinctly different from even those we serviced earlier this decade. Today, people are concerned about high quality service and predictability. They want to feel good and look good as a direct result of their salon experience. Concern about physical appearance has reached an all-time high, and people are willing to invest in themselves as long as it proves to be worth their while. Down-sizing has become the overwhelming trend for corporations, making job competition fierce, and people are living longer, more productive lives—two very good explanations for current trends in consumer tastes and spending habits.

Defining Contemporary Client Care

When you first begin modernizing your approach to client care, it is important to realize that a great care program is more than a cheerful smile. It is a planned

Good stylists who are also client-care specialists are thriving and will continue to do so well into the 21st century.

method of doing business that results in client retention, prosperity, and peace of mind. It also enables your clients to love your business and allows you to do the same. When wisely planned and faithfully practiced, a modern program of care has the power to turn business heartaches into joy and to allow everyone to experience a measure of success they have never had before. The initial planning must begin with you. In order for you to enjoy long-term success, your finished program should reflect the total of everyone's contributions.

The contemporary client care program consists of creating a beautiful environment that appeals to the five senses. Focus on salon details that add up to a positive client experience. There are many suggestions on how you can evaluate the current state of your business as well as measure your business growth as you progress to a higher state of care. The contemporary client care program also outlines a "circle of care": a planned way to directly care for your clients and staff. This portion of the program can become a beautiful blend of expertise and is the biggest area of staff ownership as it pertains to care.

A good place to begin is with a personal salon checklist.

Circle of Care

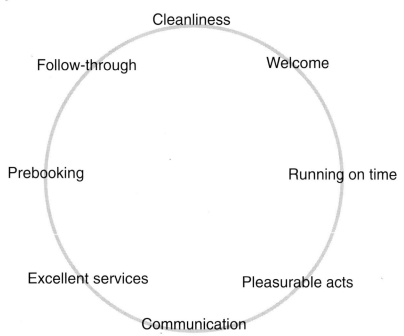

Cleanliness

Follow-through

Welcome

Prebooking

Running on time

Excellent services

Pleasurable acts

Communication

Initial Evaluation and Planning

A good place to begin is with a personal salon checklist. At this moment, how contemporary is your business? Initially this evaluation should be done completely from your point of view; other salon members can participate after your overall plan is clearer in your own mind.

Following are some questions to ask yourself:

+ How modern is my salon's approach to client care? Is it different than it was five years ago, and if so, how?
+ Do our clients receive the same care and have the same quality experience every time they enter our salon?
+ Do we have a formal client handling plan?
+ Is my approach to salon management current?
+ Do I attend management seminars regularly?

Reflecting on these questions is a great beginning in updating and changing your salon's approach to customer satisfaction. Looking through the lens of a camera is like seeing through the eyes of a client. Take some pictures of your salon at different times throughout the day. Study them carefully and, when appropriate, share them with your staff. This is a great way to convey what clients see when they are being serviced in your salon. It is also an "insightful" look at first impressions by those who are new to your establishment. What are they seeing?

The Client Within

Always remember that you, too, are a discriminating client! When you go to a restaurant, you expect to be greeted by a hostess immediately. It is her job to seat you or to give you an accurate time when a table will be available for you. If she does not appear, or the wait is longer than you were told, you know immediately that you are receiving poor service. If the poor service continues throughout your visit, how likely are you to return? Your clients judge your business in the same way you judge other businesses!

In addition to prompt care, quality service allows some businesses to prosper while others fail. Nordstrom's, for instance, has made shopping so pleasurable that their approach to business has become the standard of high excellence for major retail outlets. When you walk into their stores, you know immediately that you will be taken care of. And good experiences do not happen every once in awhile. Their great service experience is something you can look forward to every time you shop.

Salons are no different from restaurants or stores. Clients know good service from bad, and most importantly, recognize when excellence has been achieved. It is a part of everyone's job who works at your salon to make sure this always happens!

Instituting a new client care plan takes patience, practice, and love. Your staff will excel, stumble, forget, and rediscover the teachings you share with them. Good habits are a continual learning and reinforcement process. For everyone's efforts, however, you can look forward to a prosperous environment with far less trouble and more potential than you have ever experienced before.

Instituting a new client care plan takes patience, practice, and love.

THE CUSTOMER SERVICE PLAN

Many salon owners and stylists do not differentiate between "good intentions" and an actual working plan. The spirit of a sound customer service policy embodies all things commonly mentioned when talking about how to treat clients: be nice, do a good job, and many other things that filter through our industry. Although these generalities reflect a great attitude about care, they should never be mistaken for actual plans for success. A contemporary client care program is an organized way of dealing with the entire client experience. A great service is a must for satisfaction, but there are many other factors that determine whether a client will stay with a salon. Unknowingly, the salon owner may be jeopardizing stylists by alienating clients. Or, the stylists may be damaging the salon's reputation with habits that are offensive to clients. And in addition to these two key figures in the client's visit, there is a large number of other encounters that must be at *least* satisfactory.

Customizing for Success

Modernizing your approach to salon care is an individual program. Because salons are so different, plans are most successful when created on an individual basis. And, once a plan is in working order, do not be afraid to change it. You will find that some things are too rigid while others are simply not as important as you once thought. The main thing is to realize that it is alright to change your methods as long as you do not compromise your goals.

Effecting Change

Creating a business that is prepared to enter the modern age of client care takes time, training, and dedication. You are not only changing your habits and those of your entire staff, but also the routines of your clients. And although the changes will make their visits more pleasurable, they should be instituted with care. After all, clients also find comfort in familiarity. Changing a few things at a time rather than creating a shocking new environment all at once will make clients feel more at ease. By asking for and listening to their opinions, you will also make them feel they are a part of the improvements taking place.

This approach will also help your stylists remain positive. They are extremely sensitive to their clients so when client anxiety exists, it is difficult for them to have positive feelings about the situation. After all, client happiness is the primary key to retaining their clientele. If their clients are excited about the changes, however, staff members will be much more likely to support the new program with enthusiasm.

> Changing a few things at a time rather than creating a shocking new environment all at once will make clients feel more at ease.

Creating a Baseline for Care

chapter 2

HOTopic

1. Sensing your environment
2. Timing
3. Evaluating your business records
4. Implementing change at your salon

EVALUATING THE STATE OF YOUR BUSINESS

To begin formulating a custom program for your salon, you will first need to personally evaluate your business on several levels. The physical aspects of your care system can be ascertained by simply observing and conducting private walk-throughs of your operation. If you are computerized, you can conduct a salon business evaluation quite easily. You will also need to challenge yourself by working through a personal analysis—a private yardstick, so to speak, to measure the amount of commitment, capability, and love you possess as a salon owner. Finally, when the initial findings are complete, you will need to create new, realistic, and measurable goals for your business and yourself.

After you have made your initial findings, you can introduce this new project to your staff and ask for their input. When doing so, be open to suggestions. By allowing the experiences of your staff to help guide the final program, your plan will be enriched with the compiled wisdom of many qualified people who have the power to make your program a success.

When evaluating the state of your business, be sure to do the following:

✦ Evaluate physical surroundings, maintenance (procedures as well as items needing repair), and salon care plan.

✦ Evaluation salon records.

✦ Evaluate your current client care program.

+ Complete a self-evaluation.

+ Determine new, realistic, and measurable goals.

An Investment of Time

By planning ahead and setting aside time to work on your recordkeeping, you will have the pleasure of focusing on the success of your business. Your walk-throughs should be planned at various times throughout the day so that you can get an ongoing picture of your operation. Does your salon perform better on Tuesday than it does on Friday? Do you currently have a business plan to ensure that your clients receive the same great treatment every time they visit your business? If you do, is it working?

Reserve time to review the books when your salon is normally slow. Do you receive less interruptions on Tuesday than on Friday? If so, plan this portion of your evaluation accordingly. Also, when all your reports have been run, you may want to make an appointment with your accountant to receive a professional analysis of your situation.

The Salon Walk-Through

A good place to begin your evaluation is with your salon environment. As we become focused on our daily routines, it is very easy to lose sight of the total salon picture. Although a very detailed walk-through of your salon should be done with your staff, an initial check of all the nuances that make up a beautiful environment can be conducted first by you. Like your clients, do this by relying on your five senses. What do you experience?

SIGHT—Are all areas of your salon visually appealing?

SMELL—Does the salon smell good?

TOUCH—How do things feel?

TASTE—Are your refreshments delicious as well as sanitary?

SOUND—What do your clients hear while waiting and being serviced?

Make your own organized checklist of sight, smell, touch, taste, and sound. Then, move about all your areas, checking your own five senses against the environment of your salon. As you do so, always try to put yourself in the position of a client. At this point, do not worry about suggesting ways to make your salon run more smoothly. Simply put your observations in writing. These notes will give you a good starting point for improvements in the near future.

By allowing the experiences of your staff to help guide the final program, you enrich your plan with the compiled wisdom of many qualified people.

Salon Checklist

Front Desk Area

Sight

- ☐ Does it give a great first impression of beauty? Is it clean, organized, esthetically pleasing?
- ☐ Does your front desk staff visually represent fashion and beauty?
- ☐ Is it kept clean and organized throughout the day? If not, when?
- ☐ Are staff members allowed to congregate at the front desk when not busy? Are your clients being greeted by a "crowd" rather than by the salon coordinator?

Smell

- ☐ Is the air fresh as you enter the salon?
- ☐ Do you deodorize your environment with aromatherapy oils, or at the least, commercial deodorizers?

Touch

- ☐ Are your clients being greeted with a reassuring touch by those who will care for them?

Taste

- ☐ Do you offer refreshments?
- ☐ Are your refreshments kept fresh and sanitary?
- ☐ Do your refreshments cater to the contemporary tastes of your clientele? Doughnuts or low-fat baked goods? Only coffee, or do you include herbal teas? Chilled water?

Sound

- ☐ Do your salon coordinators sound genuinely pleased to see your clients?
- ☐ Are their conversations appropriate?
- ☐ Is your music appropriate in selection, quality and volume?
- ☐ Do your clients sound happy?

Service Areas

Sight

- ☐ How is your work area maintained overall?
- ☐ Are there times during the day when it appears disastrous?
- ☐ Are your chairs clean and free of product build-up?
- ☐ Do your clients sit on clumps of hair? Acrylic dust? Sticky bits of wax?

Are all areas of your salon visually appealing?

☐ Sit in various chairs throughout your work station and observe your environment through your clients' eyes. Open a few drawers while you are still sitting. What's in there? Disheveled tools, hair and globs of styling products? Or, are they organized and clean? Whatever you see, your clients will see as well.

Smell

☐ How does this area smell?

☐ Are you making every effort to provide high quality chemical services which minimize offensive odors?

☐ Do you have a ventilation system to remove smells soon after they appear?

☐ Are leftover chemical products removed immediately or do they remain in open work areas throughout the day for clients to view and smell?

Touch

☐ Does your salon have a prescribed method for protecting clients during services?

☐ Are they kept dry and comfortable at all times?

Sound

☐ Are the acoustics and music in the service areas adequate to insure good background music?

☐ Are the conversations of your service artists positive?

☐ Do your artists keep the level of their own conversations down so they won't intrude on others?

Shampoo Area

Sight

☐ Are your products organized and wiped clean?

☐ Are the products on the backbar a good representation of what you recommend for purchase in your retail area?

☐ How about your sink traps—are they full of hair? If they are, your clients will be aware of it also.

☐ Are your chairs clean and well-maintained?

☐ Any dead moths in your light fixtures?

Smell

☐ Are your towel bins emptied regularly to prevent overwhelming odors?

☐ Are chemical bottles removed immediately after use?

Touch

- ☐ When was the last time you purchased new towels? Are yours thick and luxurious or feel worn to the touch?
- ☐ Do they feel soft?
- ☐ Lay in a shampoo chair yourself for fifteen minutes or so. Are you comfortable? Do you need a neck rest?

Sound

- ☐ What do clients hear while they have their hair washed or processed? Irritating music? Nice soothing sounds?
- ☐ Are your artists quiet or talkative during this phase?

Restrooms

Sight

- ☐ Are your bathrooms attractive?
- ☐ Are your mirrors clean?
- ☐ Are your toilets maintained well?
- ☐ Are all the nooks and crannies clean?
- ☐ Do you have a plan already in place to check them throughout the day?

Smell

- ☐ How do your restrooms smell?
- ☐ Do you ventilate them at night?
- ☐ Do you have air fresheners out and available for use by clients as well as staff?

Touch

- ☐ Do you supply toilet seat covers?
- ☐ Are your paper goods in adequate supply?
- ☐ Are they of good quality?

Lab Area

Sight

- ☐ Is it visible to clients passing by? If so, what do they see? An efficient, creative area? Or, a sloppy, disheveled room? Remember, most beauty services begin in that room. Should clients be nervous or calm and reassured?

Smocks, Towels, and Sheets

Sight

- [ ] Do your cloth supplies appear to be in excellent condition? Any stains or holes? Bright or drab?
- [ ] Look at your clients in your smocks. What do you see?

Smell

- [ ] Do they smell fresh?
- [ ] Are they used only once before washing?

Touch

- [ ] Do your towels have acrylic residue or anything else that would irritate the wearer?
- [ ] Do your towels feel well-cared for?
- [ ] Are your sheets soft?
- [ ] Are your gowns stiff, or pleasant to the touch?
- [ ] Place some of your towels around your own neck, wrap yourself in your own sheets. And lastly, put on one of your salon smocks and look in the mirror. Does it help you feel good about yourself?

Other

- [ ] Do you have a regular maintenance schedule for your salon? If so, is it in writing?
- [ ] Have you designated a specific level of cleanliness for your staff? Is it in writing?
- [ ] What is the condition of your walls? Do they need painting?
- [ ] And your floors? What areas look particularly soiled?
- [ ] Are your windows clean and the sills free of dust and spider webs?
- [ ] And lastly, look between the furniture, shelving, and the walls. Any place, in fact, where dust bunnies, trash, and hair can co-mingle. Do they need a thorough cleaning?

Salon Timing

Spend some time in each of your service areas to make sure that your clients are being serviced efficiently. A wonderful service and exceptional atmosphere can be irreversibly marred if the salon does not keep within the promised appointment time. When two-hour services slip to three and appointments begin later than scheduled, clients may not complain but they may slip away quietly. The impact on the salon when a client arrives fifteen minutes late for an appointment is something everyone has experienced. The reverse is also true. We have a negative impact when we fail to take clients on time. Late beginnings affect everyone's well-being.

Salon Timing Checklist

Clients

- ☐ Are your clients always greeted at the front desk within thirty seconds of their arrival? If not, how long does it take for someone to greet them?
- ☐ Are clients' appointment times respected?
- ☐ Are clients serviced efficiently during appointments?
- ☐ Are clients being checked out within one minute of arriving at the check-out area?

Stylists

- ☐ Does your staff arrive ten to fifteen minutes before their first scheduled clients? If not, when do they arrive?
- ☐ Is your front desk prepared before the first client arrives every day?
- ☐ Do your stylists run on time?
- ☐ Do you have time parameters for services? If so, is your staff aware of them? Are the guidelines in writing?

EVALUATING YOUR SALON RECORDS

After evaluating the physical aspects of your business, you can begin evaluating your salon records. They will reveal many things. Ultimately, you will need to look at your percentage of services and retail, salon expenses, salon retention figures, as well as your current bottom-line profit. However, to trust these reports, you must first look at the source of your information: your client record cards. (Refer to Chapter Three "Computerization.")

Client Record Cards

The basis of salon information stems from good client record cards. When properly filled out, these cards allow you to know when and if clients are returning, what services they are receiving, and how much money they have spent. They also give you good indications of ways to successfully "romance" them and retain their patronage.

It is absolutely imperative to keep your records accurate and complete. Are your records always, sometimes, or never filled out? Are they complete, partially complete, or mostly blank?

> The basis of salon information stems from good client record cards.

Client Records Checklist

- [ ] Do you use a standard client profile card? If not, develop one that is appropriate for your business.
- [ ] Are your client records current? What methods are used to keep them current?
- [ ] Who controls these records? Your staff, you, or both?
- [ ] Do you carefully detail haircut appointments as well as chemical services?
- [ ] Randomly check your profile cards for everyone visiting on a given day. Are they completely filled out? Do this several times throughout one month. Are Tuesday's records better than Friday's?
- [ ] If computerized, run a client list and randomly select a few names. Compare them to the actual forms your clients have filled out. Are your client records being input correctly?
- [ ] Run a client list for everyone who has visited your salon during the last three months. Are there blank spots where addresses and telephone numbers should be? Is there any other information missing?
- [ ] Run a client list by individual stylist. Do some have unusual amounts of blank spaces where addresses and telephone numbers should be?
- [ ] How many postings have been made under the catch-all name of "salon client"? This generic name should only refer to one-time clients who are visiting from out of town, or to walk-ins who purchase retail and decline to fill out a card.

After you have evaluated the condition of your client cards, check your books during times when your business is closed. Compare the names on your books against the names in your computer. Are they being spelled properly? If not, your entire salon evaluation will be faulty. Names on the books are generally transferred to service tickets. Service tickets are then input into the computer, dispersing information about clients, services, and payroll. Accuracy can not be stressed enough!

Service Tickets

Service tickets tell a wealth of information about a client. It's a good idea to take the time to check for spellings, legibility, and accuracy of information on as many service tickets as you can for a period of a month or more. This will give you a good sense of whether you can rely on any information you have up to that point, give it partial credence, or have complete faith in what it says.

Also, make sure that the service options listed on the ticket are current. If you have added waxing but are still putting it under "other," consider adding it as a separate category. This will help you ascertain later whether particular services are generating enough capital to warrant promotions or greater capital investment by the salon.

Begin by running several different client reports. How many perms and colors have you done within the last month? How many within the last quarter? How many extra services were performed? How many haircuts were completed?

Retail sales information also originates with the service ticket. Run a retail report to determine how active your stock is. Products that remain on the shelf longer than four weeks are tying up money that could be used to otherwise enhance your business. Work with your staff at a later date to determine why products are not moving. For now, check your reports. If your program breaks down your sales by A (most active), B, C, and D (dead) activity, by all means utilize this information in your decision-making.

Salon Activity Checklist

- ☐ Determine the service habits of clients. How many services have been performed over the last month? How many over the last quarter? What kind of services have been performed?
- ☐ Run these same reports by stylists.
- ☐ Figure the total retail purchases.
- ☐ Which of your products are moving (sold within the last four weeks)?
- ☐ Which of your products are stagnant (not sold within the last four weeks)?
- ☐ How long do clients remain with your salon? Are your files filled with inactive cards? If so, how many?

The information gathered by completing the salon activity checklist will be inaccurate if your service tickets and client record cards are incomplete or not current. However, you can still use the information as a baseline for the future growth of your records. Check service tickets and client record cards in three months to see if the information is more accurate, more complete, and current. Mark your own progress, and do not forget to give yourself a pat on the back. Keeping good records is not a flashy accomplishment, but it is every bit as important as a great cut or busy day. In the long run, accurate records may be even more important.

And once you have accurate information, you can track client retention, romance your patrons with thank-yous, and help all of your stylists nurture their own success.

Checking the Percentages

Checking the percentages of performance by your salon is also a necessary step before goals for better performance can be contemplated. Your software program should have easy-to-read graphs for sales, services, and individual stylists' records. If it does not, the profit and loss statement (P&L) provided by your accountant should contain much of this information. Again, your

> Products that remain on the shelf longer than four weeks are tying up money that could be used to otherwise enhance your business.

records must be accurate and up-to-date for this information to have any validity. If you have found that your recordkeeping needs improvement, wait until you have your postings perfected for at least three months before utilizing these figures as a basis for future improvements of your business.

Client Retention

The ability to track client retention via computer is an excellent capability. As an automated salon, give yourself at least six months to perfect your records and then begin the task of tracking client retention. This should give the majority of your clients ample opportunity to return to your salon at least three times. Doing this portion of your evaluation too early can create inaccurate and often disturbing results. For instance, a report may indicate that a stylist has an extremely low retention rate simply because clients were continually inputted in the computer program under various spellings, each one indicating a new person who usually did not return. Good guidelines for client retention are:

◆ 85% request rate by established clientele.

◆ 10% new clients (5% supplied by the stylist and 5% supplied by the salon).

◆ 5% salon clients who normally go to another stylist or simply have no stylist preference.

Percentage of Services

There are three general guidelines for a healthy mix of salon services and retail. (These can be more accurately evaluated after your client/service records have been complete for ninety days or more.) If your salon is close to these sales percentages, you already have a healthy mix of basic business which will be invaluable in creating a successful salon!

Service/Retail	Sales Percentage
Haircuts/styles	55% or less
Chemical services	45% or more
Retail sales	18% or more

After you have determined how your salon is performing as a whole, run the same information by stylist. What are their individual percentages? Are they higher or lower than the salon norm? Do you have a few stylists who are carrying many? Or, does your staff simply need a larger client base?

Profit vs. Expenses

Evaluating this area is often the most painful thing a salon owner can do. After all, doesn't hard work equate to good income? Maybe if you are behind the chair, but *running* an entire salon has no guarantees. If your profit and loss statement does not reflect the time and energy you have devoted to your business, the wisest thing you can do is to become proactive in changing the situation.

In order to provide the comforts your clients deserve, you will need to review your overall expenditures and eliminate waste wherever possible. In a very small salon, it is not unusual to discover $1,000 a month or more simply being squandered, sometimes pennies at a time! A general guideline for bottom line percentages on your profit and loss statement are as follows:

+ *Payroll*—30%-35% maximum. This includes commission stylists, front desk employees, management staff, and a shop maid. Note: These percentages do not apply to a booth rental salon.
+ *Service supplies*—2%-5% maximum.
+ *Shop supplies* (office and general salon)—1% or less.
+ *Rent*—10-12% maximum.
+ *Advertising* and *promotion*—3% maximum.
+ *Utilities*, including telephone—1%.

This is also a good time to contact your accountant. Bringing your records to a professional can save you endless hours of paperwork by making sure you collect data that truly counts for your business. Share your plans for a more contemporary care system and invite suggestions for ways to better assemble your records. Then within three months, also bring your new, improved records to the accountant for a re-appraisal. With this more accurate information, ask for suggestions on ways to save money, as well as make more dollars through cost management strategies.

> In a very small salon, it is not unusual to discover $1,000 a month or more simply being squandered, sometimes pennies at a time!

Self-Evaluation

While running a salon is a difficult job, it is an absolutely impossible job if the salon owner does not love the business. Before investing time and energy into a new project, take a moment and question your motivations. Are you in the salon business because you feel there is money to be made there? Are you really in love with owning and running a salon? It takes more passion to build a great business than it does to perfect artistic skills. And, like all other aspects of the beauty business, it requires even more interest to do it well.

The contemporary client care program will never become something that will not require your attention. But, it will give you a greater chance to satisfy a burning desire to own a successful business. One that performs for you and provides security for your associates by allowing you to concentrate on a bright business future rather than being consumed by the woes of today.

But for all of this to come true, you have got to love what you do and show that love by being devoted to learning, practicing and sharing the best knowledge available. Owning a salon can be the highest point of your life or your lowest ebb. It is such a flamboyant, fast-paced enterprise that both of these emotions can even be experienced within the same day—especially if you have not yet committed to investing in this program of care.

Professional Checklist

Ask yourself these important personal questions and reflect on your answers when developing your contemporary client care program:

- ☐ How do you really feel about your business? Are you ecstatic or sorry that you are a salon owner?
- ☐ Do you trust yourself with your future as well as the future of your staff? Do you trust your employees with your future?
- ☐ Do you feel satisfied with your salon?
- ☐ Are you close to the clients of your salon?
- ☐ Are you good about maintaining current salon books?
- ☐ Do you frequently study your salon records or do you fear and ignore them?
- ☐ Do you lead your salon through inspiration? If not, how do you do it?
- ☐ Are you education driven? Are you committed to promoting continuing education among your staff?
- ☐ How many management courses do you attend per year?
- ☐ How many artistic seminars do you attend per year?
- ☐ Are you computer automated?
- ☐ Do you use your software programs wisely?
- ☐ Is your business growing?
- ☐ Is your profit increasing with your growth?
- ☐ Are you "fluent" in salon reports? Do you understand graphs and charts?
- ☐ Are you "fluent" in accounting reports? Can you read a P&L statement?
- ☐ Is your business steady? Are your chairs full?
- ☐ Are your stylists' books built?
- ☐ Do you really know if your staff is happy?
- ☐ Are you artistically driven? If you are, is this creative force shared with your staff? How?
- ☐ While servicing clients, do you personally have clean habits?
- ☐ Are you an example of model behavior?
- ☐ Does your staff respect you?

- ☐ Do you have regular staff meetings? Do you have good attendance at your staff meetings? Are your meetings informative, positive, and well planned?
- ☐ Are you groomed to reflect fashion trends?
- ☐ If you had it to do over, what would you do differently?
- ☐ Do you have balance in your life, including, work, play, and creative expression?
- ☐ Are you professionally satisfied? Explain.
- ☐ Do you have the support of your family, or does the time spent managing your business create hardships in your relationships?
- ☐ Name the five most important things in your life in their order of importance. Is your salon business among the top five? Are you successful with the other four?
- ☐ Make two lists, one for the positive aspects of your business, and one for the negative aspects of your business. Will a more contemporary client care system help eliminate some of the drawbacks you are experiencing? Will it accentuate the positive? If so, how?
- ☐ Do you regularly set vivid, specific goals? Do you follow through with your goals? Do you accomplish them? Name three goals you have accomplished recently.
- ☐ What are your plans for the upcoming year?
- ☐ What are your plans for the next five years?
- ☐ Do you have plans for another career?

Do you have balance in your life, including, work, play, and creative expression?

IMPLEMENTING THE FIRST CHANGES

The information you have gathered by completing the previous checklists will allow you to soon create your own "circle of care" for your clients. By organizing your salon records, you are able to reward, contact, and retrieve those who use your services. And, after conducting walk-throughs and observing your people, you also have at least a general idea of what needs to be done to improve the quality and consistency of the client experience. Your next step will be to begin implementing changes that affect your own performance and that of your front desk. It is also a great time to learn what your clients think of your salon, receive their suggestions for improvements and act on those which will make their time in your business positive and profitable. Above all, begin sharing your efforts with your staff. Let them know that you are working towards a better business environment for everyone who has invested time and effort in your salon.

chapter 3

Computerization

HOTopic

1. Automated system of care
2. Specialty salon software
3. Creating a database for service

GATHERING INFORMATION

Before changing anything about your salon, evaluating the business from top to bottom is a very important step. Not only do you need to know the general state of your business before planning a new program, you also must learn detailed information about every area that impacts your bottom line.

Computers serve many functions in the salon, including tracking inventory and quickly processing payroll. But their greatest asset is the ability to help you retain your clients. Computers do this by providing a vivid picture of your business, helping you market your goods and services, providing an efficient checkout procedure, plus supplying accurate reports on demand. Once your salon is computerized (automated), you will be ready to upgrade by creating a contemporary method of care.

Be patient with yourself, as well as others, while you are instituting this portion of your program, and do not expect results overnight. In fact, it will take several months for you to accumulate enough information to accurately analyze your situation, and probably even longer to acclimate everyone to the changes needed to make the program a success.

Entering the world of computerization can be mildly difficult for some and exasperating for others. Indeed, while you are still learning to load programs and run reports, your computer may even seem to take on a personality all its own! But these aspects will pass while other more positive things will not. Your computer will continue to fascinate you and give you new and improved information. Most problems will disappear with education and simple exposure to the process. The problems that will inevitably crop up in the future will be handled with greater ease due to your ever-growing expertise.

Delegating Time

While salon software has become sophisticated, it is still simple to use. It does not take an accountant or a computer whiz to operate the programs. But it will always require time. And while a computer can generate a report quickly, it must have accurate, current information in order to be of any value. This can only be accomplished if you set time aside to input new information on a regular basis.

It is important not to expand your work hours to accomplish this. Your workload is most likely already excessive and any additional time dedication would be unreasonable. Instead, think delegation. What responsibilities can you delegate to others so that you can perform this critical function? Or, who can you hire to do it for you? If you hire someone, check their work frequently and thoroughly and be sure to give the person explicit directions on how you want your postings to be handled. Always check their input at least once a week—other people will never take your business as seriously as you do.

SOFTWARE FOR SERVICE

Purchasing your first computer, dedicating yourself to learning an entirely new set of skills, and re-orienting those who come in contact with your salon is a very large project. You may experience times when you ask yourself, "Why did I ever think we should do this?" Your staff, perhaps resistant to change, might even be upset initially because of the loss of their familiar routine. Even your clients may require some hand-holding.

And, of course, there is you, the salon owner, who is helping others while trying to understand the process yourself. With the right guidance, however, any computer-related stumbling blocks you may experience will quickly dissipate as your skill level rises. In fact, you can become top-notch with your programs in a relatively short period of time. Classes are often available with the purchase of a computer and most salon software companies offer special instruction for their program users. Help will always be available to you when needed, especially if you shop smart before committing to the purchase of this valuable piece of equipment. Shopping for education is just as important as insisting on the best possible price!

Once up and running, your computer will check out clients more efficiently and while doing this, it will also record all the services your clients received that day, the total dollars spent, and when clients are due to return. The information

Computers serve many functions in the salon, including tracking inventory and quickly processing payroll.

will also be distributed automatically to your salon sales records. Generated by specialized salon programs, these records can make your client care system absolutely top-notch. In addition to keeping track of product sales and services, your computer can also be utilized as a powerful marketing tool to enhance your clients' salon experience. The list of capabilities does not stop here. It is actually the beginning of a lengthy menu of functions and benefits that will help make your salon stable, prosperous, and busy.

Computer Capabilities

In addition to a variety of other functions, your salon computer is capable of:

- ✦ Producing a report that includes clients' addresses and telephone numbers.
- ✦ Giving needed information to point out clients who are overdue for visits.
- ✦ Printing thank-you notes, gift certificates, and salon newsletters.
- ✦ Supplying information that may be used for general, as well as specific, promotions (products or services).
- ✦ Generating in-house signage and flyers.
- ✦ Addressing post cards and envelopes.
- ✦ Separating your clients by salon artist for individual promotions.
- ✦ Separating your clients by purchase preferences for special promotions.
- ✦ Keeping vital information that will allow you to stay in touch with your clients for a variety of reasons.
- ✦ Tracking results of promotions and other marketing activities.
- ✦ Tracking retention rate of salon artists as well as your business overall.

In addition to keeping track of product sales and services, your computer can also be utilized as a powerful marketing tool to enhance your clients' salon experience.

Hardware/Software Differences

Written for this book by Tom Maple, Salon Transcripts.

There is often confusion about the difference between hardware and software. One analogy could be a stereo: The hardware in a stereo system includes the CD player, amplifier, and speakers; the software is the music recorded on the cassettes or CDs (not the cassettes or CDs themselves but *music recorded on them*). The music can be played on a cheap stereo or an expensive one. An expensive stereo will make the music sound better but unless one has the music they like to hear, no stereo will be pleasing.

With a computer system, the hardware consists of a keyboard, mouse, monitor, printer, disk drive, CD drive, hard drive, and the processing unit. The software is the programs recorded on diskettes, CDs, or the hard drive.

Order of Implementation

In order to learn how to "walk before you run," start by entering your client cards in the computer. By having your client data computerized, you will be able to promote your salon to your current clientele. After mastering the client database, enter the daily sales tickets. From this, all other areas of the system are updated. This is where the old adage "garbage in, garbage out" applies most. If it is not done correctly, nothing else in the system will be right. Once these steps are accomplished, some of the more "bean counting" aspects of computerization such as inventory and payroll can be implemented.

The Missing Records Story

Not long ago a, businesswoman in Southern California grew weary of posting her own books. So, she selected a good employee with great aptitude for the computer and had her input daily sales receipts and process payroll. No one complained that their check was wrong and all the figures added up at the end of the week. Everything seemed perfect!

One month and 2,000 clients later, the owner decided to take a peek at her monthly client records. She discovered, despite providing her employees with explicit training, that twelve hundred of the clients who had visited that month were put under the catch-all category of "salon client" rather than by their individual names. Nearly a month of individual client records had gone unrecorded! The clients in question were not given credit for their visits; client retention records by stylists and the salon as a whole were lost and retail and service sales records on individual customers during that period were gone for good.

When the owner asked why this had happened, the employee simply said, "Checking on all those names took too long. 'Salon Client' is much faster. And besides, I don't have time to gather up all that information."

Looking back on it later, the owner realized that the real problem was not the time spent doing these daily tasks, but rather the fact that she had not delegated other responsibilities so that she could have computer time without adding extra hours to her work week. (How much easier it would have been for someone else to count paper towels and cups!) The owner who learned a valuable lesson that day was "yours truly." It is nice to note, however, that the end had a very positive result: My records became as sacred as my checkbook and from that day forward, they both received the best of care!

Beauty Industry Software

While there are many different software programs you can purchase for your computer, the beauty industry provides specialized software packages that meet the specific needs of salons. By utilizing these programs, you are empowering yourself and your staff with the ability to give every client the ultimate experience of great care. Software is more than counting. It is also an essential tool when creating a contemporary client care system.

Choosing a Report System

When choosing a system for your business, make sure to study carefully the reports they produce. Are they easy to read and laid out in a clear and concise manner? Do they provide all the information you need to create a superb client care system?

And, especially in the first year of computerization, be sure to consider what type of technical support you can expect from your computer and its software. All software (programs) and hardware (equipment) companies work differently. Some offer 800 numbers while others want you to call across the continent on your dime. There are only a few companies with adequate technical staff to care for your needs promptly, with many taking several hours and sometimes even days to respond to your call.

Always read the manuals for the equipment and programs. Are they written in a clear and concise manner? Would you be able to solve simple problems or learn basic techniques from these books? If the answer is "yes," then you have already gained a measure of independence. Calling a hotline can be expensive and time consuming, but a guide that offers in-depth, understandable information may be referenced in a matter of minutes. It will also save both you and the computer company unneeded calls for assistance.

> Especially in the first year of computerization, be sure to consider what type of technical support you can expect from your computer and its software.

COMPUTERIZED CLIENT INFORMATION

With regular input and accurate spelling of names, you will be able to learn several things about your clients and staff. The following are report examples of computer printouts that can be made available to everyone in your salon.

The Client Questionnaire

Every client in your salon, whether new or existing, should complete a client questionnaire. This information will enable you to care for them in countless ways. For example, marketing/client care information taken from this questionnaire will ultimately provide you with:

- ✦ An individual client list for the stylist
- ✦ A marketable client base for the salon
- ✦ What products they prefer
- ✦ What services they have had in the past

CLIENT QUESTIONNAIRE

First Name _____ Middle Initial _____ Today's Date _____

Last Name _____

Address _____

City _____ State _____ Zip _____

Home Ph. _____ Work _____

Birthday: ____ / ____ / ____

Occupation: _____ Stylist: _____

How did you hear of our salon? _____ D/L No. _____

Date of last visit (if any): ____ / ____ / ____ Service(s) today: _____

Please answer the following questions to receive your personalized prescription:

HAIR LENGTH
- [ ] 0 to 2 inches
- [ ] 3 to 4 inches
- [ ] 5 to 7 inches
- [ ] 8 to 12 inches
- [ ] Over 12 inches

HAIR TEXTURE
- [ ] Very fine
- [ ] Fine
- [ ] Medium
- [ ] Coarse

SCALP CONDITION
- [ ] Dry
- [ ] Oily
- [ ] Dandruff/Itching
- [ ] Normal

HAIR CONDITION
- [ ] Dry
- [ ] Humidity causes frizzing
- [ ] Breaking
- [ ] Split ends
- [ ] Style readily falls
- [ ] No damage evident

STYLING METHOD
- [ ] Blow-dryer
- [ ] Curling iron/ hot rollers
- [ ] Roller set
- [ ] Wet look
- [ ] Air dry

HAIR SERVICE TODAY
- [ ] Haircut
- [ ] Perm
- [ ] Bleach/Tint
- [ ] Weaving
- [ ] Cellophane
- [ ] Relaxer
- [ ] Not Sure

I'VE HAD A
- [ ] Perm
- [ ] Bleach/Tint
- [ ] Weaving/Highlights
- [ ] Cellophane
- [ ] Relaxer
- [ ] No chemical service

OTHER CONDITIONS
- [ ] Prescribed medecine
- [ ] Birth control pills
- [ ] Hard water
- [ ] Pool or jacuzzi
- [ ] Sun exposure
- [ ] Vitamins/Caffeine
- [ ] None of the above

FOR STYLING AID, I LIKE
- [ ] Light hold
- [ ] Medium hold
- [ ] Firm hold
- [ ] No preference

I PREFER MOUSSE
- [ ] Yes
- [ ] No
- [ ] No preference

I CONDITION MY HAIR
- [ ] Daily
- [ ] Twice a week
- [ ] Weekly
- [ ] Monthly
- [ ] Never

CONDITIONER(S) USED
- [ ] Moisturizer
- [ ] Protein reconstructor
- [ ] After-shampoo rinse
- [ ] Leave-in conditioner
- [ ] Hot oil treatment

LAST PERM
- [ ] 4 weeks ago or less
- [ ] 6 weeks ago
- [ ] 2 months ago
- [ ] 3 months ago
- [ ] Longer

DURING LAST PERM
- [ ] Sat under dryer/lamps
- [ ] Didn't use dryer/lamps

LAST BLEACH/TINT/WEAVE
- [ ] 2 weeks ago or less
- [ ] 4 weeks ago
- [ ] 6 weeks ago
- [ ] 2 months ago
- [ ] Longer

- How they found your salon and/or their stylist
- The date they first came to your salon
- Their birthday
- Whether they are married

The client questionnaire is, without a doubt, the most valuable source of information your salon can possess. The information gathered from this form will allow you to count, "romance," and reward all clients who have entrusted their goodwill to your salon. And, equally as beautiful is the fact that, once this information is inputted into your computer, it will automatically sort, report, and print nearly any combination of information you wish to see.

Salon Transcripts Client Selection					
Name	**Address**	**City**	**Zip**	**Eve Phone**	**Day Phone**
Biondi, Celeste 01/13/68	567 Main St.	Los Angeles	91601	555-1234	555-1234
Carson, Kim 01/01/49	567 Main St.	Los Angeles	91601	555-1234	555-1234
Granger, Pat 01/05/45	567 Main St.	Los Angeles	91601	555-1234	555-1234
Kelley, Joyce 01/01/45	567 Main St.	Los Angeles	91601	555-1234	555-1234
Lara, Alicia 01/01/48	567 Main St.	Los Angeles	91601	555-1234	555-1234
Ward, Rosalee 01/25/48	567 Main St.	Los Angeles	91601	555-1234	555-1234
Weatherly, Mary 01/01/49	567 Main St.	Los Angeles	91601	555-1234	555-1234

7 clients selected or 4.79% of your clients.
Birthdate in 1/0/00

Service/Retail Tickets

Another resource you will have when using salon software is the information from the service/retail ticket filled out at the end of each visit. From this ticket, you know who came in, what services and products they purchased, and who took care of them that day. Notice how each price is broken out, the totals are separated for services and products, and then combined as a grand total at the bottom of the slip. Information gleaned from the service ticket will provide you with:

Salon Name

Appointment Time _____ Date _____

First Name _____

Last Name _____

Stylist's Name _____

Sty.	Service	Price	Retail Ticket		
			Qty.	Stock #	Price
			Sales SUBTOTAL		
			Sales TAX		
			Retail TOTAL		

Service Total $ _____

Retail Total $ _____

TOTAL $ _____

Service _____%Discount   Retail _____%Discount

☐ Male   ☐ Female
☐ Regular Req. ☐ New Request
☐ Salon Client ☐ Walk-in
☐ Cash   ☐ American Express
☐ Check   ☐ Gift
☐ MasterCard   ☐ Preferred Customer
☐ VISA   ☐ Charge Acct.

- A current client list for the stylist
- A marketable client base for the salon
- The value of each client in terms of money spent during a specific time at your salon
- Services they are receiving
- Services they are not receiving
- Discontinued services
- Services they have added
- How often they come to your salon
- What products they prefer
- How they found your salon and/or their stylist
- Method of payment

SALON ANALYSIS

One of the best aspects of a good salon software program is the ability to measure and report the performance of your salon and your stylists during any given time period. (See Fig. 3-1, pg. 33, for an example.) By completing a salon analysis, you will learn:

- Total amount of money earned
- Amount of money earned on individual services
- Amount of money earned on individual products
- Total amount of money earned on products
- Percentage of these services or products as it relates to your total dollar intake
- Amount of regular business your salon enjoys
- Amount of new clientele your salon is generating and some information about how they found you
- Percentage of your retail sales to service dollars
- Average service ticket dollar amount
- Average number of services per client

Given this information, you can find out what areas are doing well and which need your attention. These figures can give everyone a starting point to create concrete goals for improvement and success. And, just as important, these reports can be run on an individual basis, giving you the same analysis for each member of your staff.

Salon Transcripts
Sales Analysis

SALON 02/01/96-02/07/96

Service	Sales	#	Avg	%
Color				
Cellophane	652.50	22	29.66	12.4
Color	659.75	19	34.72	12.5
Dbl. Process	225.00	5	45.00	4.3
Highlights	195.00	3	65.00	3.7
Color subtotal	1,732.25	49	35.35	32.9
Cut/Style				
Female Cut	600.00	24	25.00	11.4
Male Cut	278.00	14	19.86	5.3
Styling	801.00	67	11.96	15.2
Cut/Style subtotal	1,679.00	105	15.99	31.9
Nails				
Nails	15.00	1	15.00	0.3
Nails subtotal	15.00	1	15.00	0.3
Other				
Condition	429.00	36	11.92	8.2
Other subtotal	429.00	36	11.92	8.2
Perm				
Perm	1,260.00	21	60.00	24.0
Prt. Perm	75.00	3	25.00	1.4
Perm subtotal	1,335.00	24	55.62	25.4
Skin Care				
Makeup	70.00	2	35.00	1.3
Skin Care subtotal	70.00	2	35.00	1.3
TOTAL SERVICE	**5,260.25**	**217**	**24.24**	
Retail	861.50	46	18.73	16.4
less returns	-40.00	2	-20.00	
Net Retail	**821.50**	**44**	**18.67**	

Net Retail is 13.5% of Total Sales

Client Type	#Clients	%	Srvc$	Avg Srvc	#Srvc/clnt
Regular Requests	76	81.7	4,438.25	58.40	2.4
Salon Clients	3	3.2	173.00	57.67	2.3
New Requests	10	10.8	498.00	49.80	2.1
Walk-ins	4	4.3	151.00	37.75	1.5
Total Clients	**93**		**5,260.25**	**56.56**	**2.3**
Retail Clients	30	32.2			1.5

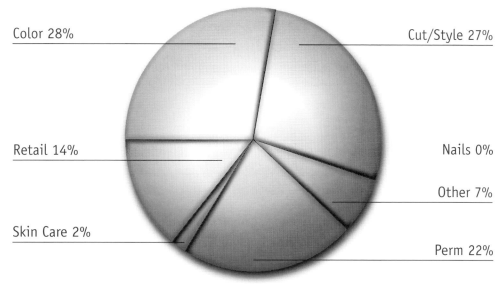

Color 28%

Cut/Style 27%

Retail 14%

Nails 0%

Other 7%

Skin Care 2%

Perm 22%

Figure 3-1
Salon Analysis

Client Retention

In order to measure the success of your client care system, your salon must know its overall client retention rate plus the retention figures of every stylist on your staff. To accurately obtain this information, it is imperative that every client be properly logged into your computer records so that their visits are accurately recorded. The results of client retention reports often prove to be the most surprising! This report will reveal:

✦ How many of your clients stay with your salon

✦ How many of your clients do not stay

✦ Which stylists are retaining 85% or more of their clients

✦ Who is not retaining 85% or more of their clients

✦ How many new clients each stylist is receiving

✦ How many new clients your salon generates

Salon Transcripts									
Client Retention									
4/1/98-7/31/98									
Employee	#New	One Time		Two Time		Emp Retain		Salon Retain	
Elliot Hamlin	20	16	80.0%	2	10.0%	0	0.0%	2	10.0%
Jeanine A. Edwards	10	7	70.0%	2	20.0%	0	0.0%	1	10.0%
Loretta M. Francis	12	6	50.0%	5	41.7%	0	0.0%	1	8.3%
Mark D. Palmquist	10	10	100.0%	0	0.0%	0	0.0%	0	0.0%
Ruth Ann Garcia	7	7	100.00%	0	0.0%	0	0.0%	0	0.0%
Renee J. Pipkin	15	8	53.3%	4	26.7%	0	0.0%	3	20.0%
Salon Total	74	54	73.0%	13	17.6%	0	0.0%	7	9.5%

With this information, you will have a much firmer grip on the reality of your business performance. And this report, along with your salon analysis, will also give you a sound basis for goals for greater client care and be a tool to measure your progress.

Client Database

Unlike most client lists that are done manually, a computerized list can tell you, at a glance:

- ✦ The total number of clients you service
- ✦ Date of last service
- ✦ Who is missing
- ✦ Clients in descending order of dollars spent at your salon
- ✦ Types of services
- ✦ Much more

<table>
<tr><td colspan="5" align="center">Salon Transcripts
Client File</td></tr>
<tr><td>Name</td><td>Address</td><td>City/St/Zip</td><td>Day/Eve</td><td>Other/Birth</td></tr>
<tr><td>Adelezzi, Cyndi</td><td>567 Main St.</td><td>Los Angeles 91423</td><td>555-1234</td><td>2/26/42</td></tr>
<tr><td>Agnos, Irene</td><td>567 Main St.</td><td></td><td></td><td>2/23/75</td></tr>
<tr><td>Akin, Kevin</td><td>567 Main St.</td><td>Los Angeles 91423</td><td>555-1234</td><td>2/3/47</td></tr>
<tr><td>Alais, Dennis</td><td>567 Main St.</td><td></td><td></td><td>8/5/53</td></tr>
<tr><td>Bagley, Elyse</td><td>567 Main St.</td><td>Los Angeles 91423</td><td>555-1234</td><td>11/9/49</td></tr>
<tr><td>Barajas, Lucinda</td><td>567 Main St.</td><td>Los Angeles 91423</td><td></td><td></td></tr>
<tr><td>Barajas, Maria</td><td>567 Main St.</td><td>Los Angeles 91423</td><td></td><td>2/27/59</td></tr>
<tr><td>Baumann, Jerome</td><td>567 Main St.</td><td>Los Angeles 91423</td><td>555-1234</td><td>8/12/47</td></tr>
<tr><td>Bell, Carol</td><td>567 Main St.</td><td>Los Angeles 91423</td><td>555-1234</td><td>8/6/49</td></tr>
<tr><td>Bennett, Kathy</td><td>567 Main St.</td><td></td><td></td><td></td></tr>
<tr><td>Biondi, Heather</td><td>567 Main St.</td><td>Los Angeles 91423</td><td>555-1234</td><td>2/3/55</td></tr>
<tr><td>Blakeley, Chuck</td><td>567 Main St.</td><td>Los Angeles 91423</td><td>555-1234</td><td>2/24/72</td></tr>
<tr><td>Bontrager, Carol</td><td>567 Main St.</td><td>Los Angeles 91423</td><td></td><td>8/5/72</td></tr>
<tr><td>Bradley, Patty</td><td>567 Main St.</td><td>Los Angeles 91423</td><td>555-1234</td><td>2/4/67</td></tr>
<tr><td>Brewer, Mark</td><td>567 Main St.</td><td>Los Angeles 91423</td><td>555-1234</td><td>2/27/42</td></tr>
<tr><td>Brittain, Sandy</td><td>567 Main St.</td><td>Los Angeles 91423</td><td></td><td>2/25/48</td></tr>
<tr><td>Brodie, Karen</td><td>567 Main St.</td><td>Los Angeles 91423</td><td>555-1234</td><td>2/5/53</td></tr>
<tr><td>Brosier, Sarah</td><td>567 Main St.</td><td>Los Angeles 91423</td><td>555-1234</td><td>2/23/70</td></tr>
</table>

Salon Transcripts
Client Selection

Name	Address	City	Zip	EvePhn	DayPhn
Agnos, Irene	567 Main St.	Los Angeles	91542		
Akin, Kevin	567 Main St.	Los Angeles	91542	555-1234	
Bagley, Elyse	567 Main St.	Los Angeles	91542	555-1234	555-1234
Balavage, Monica	567 Main St.	Los Angeles	91542	555-1234	555-1234
Curry, Ken	567 Main St.	Los Angeles	91542	555-1234	555-1234
Daley, Sue					
Dana, Deane	567 Main St.	Los Angeles	91542	555-1234	555-1234
Ellison, Jonathan	567 Main St.	Los Angeles	91542		
Fong, Curtis	567 Main St.	Los Angeles	91542	555-1234	555-1234
Genco, Jane	567 Main St.	Los Angeles	91542	555-1234	
Gosset, Loretta	567 Main St.	Los Angeles	91542		
Hafron, Andrea	567 Main St.	Los Angeles	91542	555-1234	
Handlen, Pam	567 Main St.	Los Angeles	91542		
Ikesaki, Lori	567 Main St.	Los Angeles	91542	555-1234	
Kay, Ursula	567 Main St.	Los Angeles	91542	555-1234	555-1234
Knudsen, Carol	567 Main St.	Los Angeles	91542	555-1234	555-1234
Lee, James	567 Main St.	Los Angeles	91542	555-1234	555-1234
Lewis, Christine	567 Main St.	Los Angeles	91542	555-1234	
MacBride, Robert	567 Main St.	Los Angeles	91542	555-1234	
Mathews, Kelly	567 Main St.	Los Angeles	91542	555-1234	
Moeller, Alice	567 Main St.	Los Angeles	91542	555-1234	555-1234
Nakamura, Joni	567 Main St.	Los Angeles	91542	555-1234	
Nootenboom, Michelle	567 Main St.	Los Angeles	91542	555-1234	
Orchard, Rebecca	567 Main St.	Los Angeles	91542	555-1234	
Pfiefer, Betty	567 Main St.	Los Angeles	91542	555-1234	555-1234
Ross, Shannon	567 Main St.	Los Angeles	91542	555-1234	
Schafer, Barry	567 Main St.	Los Angeles	91542	555-1234	555-1234
Tomita, Lisa	567 Main St.	Los Angeles	91542		
Ward, Rosalee	567 Main St.	Los Angeles	91542	555-1234	555-1234
Young, Kathy	567 Main St.	Los Angeles	91542	555-1234	555-1234

30 clients selected or 13.57% of your clients.
Emp/Service, emp:Sandra Smith

With this knowledge, you can send automated mailers with little effort and less expense, have a call sheet to let clients know of special events, and a reward system for those who remain loyal to your business.

CREATING A COMPLETE DATABASE

A complete list of all clients who come to your salon is valuable for overall marketing purposes. This list can be put together as an entire database, or be separated by stylist. Because the information is so clearly laid out, it is obvious when addresses and telephone numbers are missing. If tracked carefully, missing information can be filled in at the client's next visit to your salon.

Running a separate list for stylists not only gives them a client database for their records, it also allows you to pinpoint their missing clients, individually promote extra services, and employ other marketing possibilities to bolster their earnings as well as your own.

By knowing the top 20% of your clients in terms of spending power, you can more effectively reward their investment in your services and products. Your top 20% deserve special treats (extra services), private sales, and more. The computer will easily tell you in any given time frame who has turned "platinum."

You can also sort out your clients by services and the date of last service. By tracking these reports, you not only know which services your clients now enjoy, but also which ones you will want to introduce in the future. And, if perms, for instance, have been done on particular clients but they have not returned for another in many months, you can send incentives to be used toward their next perm appointment at your salon.

Checking for Accuracy

By running out a fresh client list on a monthly basis, you not only catch missing information right away, but discover and discard "ghosts." Ghost clients are those who are incorrectly entered into your computer by way of improper spelling of a name.

For example, in this list, Rosemary Ahrens has also been listed as Rose Ahrens, Rosemary Erins, Rose Arons, and Rosemary Aaron.

If you do not ask clients how they spell their names, misspellings will occur frequently in your client database. When this happens, the retention rates of your stylists appear lower than they actually are, clients cannot be accurately tracked for missing/return incentives, and your stylists' records erroneously show that multiple new clients have been provided for them. Also, the value of individual clients cannot be accurately assessed and bad entries can dramatically inflate your total client database.

By knowing the top 20% of your clients' spending power, you can more effectively reward their investment.

Salon Transcripts
Client Selection

Name	Address	City	Zip	EvePhn	DayPhn
Aaron, Rosemary					
Adelizzi, Cyndi	567 Main St.	Los Angeles	91423	555-1234	555-1234
Ahrens, Rose	567 Main St.	Los Angeles	91423		
Ahrens, Rosemary	567 Main St.	Los Angeles	91423	555-1234	555-1234
Akers, Sandy					
Arons, Rose	567 Main St.	Los Angeles	91423	555-1234	
Bagley, Elise	567 Main St.	Los Angeles	91423	555-1234	555-1234
Balavage, Monica	567 Main St.	Los Angeles	91423	555-1234	555-1234
Biondi, Heather	567 Main St.	Los Angeles	91423	555-1234	555-1234
Erins, Rosemary	567 Main St.	Los Angeles	91423		
Ferguson, Sherilyn	567 Main St.	Los Angeles	91423	555-1234	
Genco, Jane	567 Main St.	Los Angeles	91423	555-1234	
Gota, Nancy	567 Main St.	Los Angeles	91423	555-1234	555-1234
Grassell, Rita	567 Main St.	Los Angeles	91423	555-1234	555-1234
Gross, Linda	567 Main St.	Los Angeles	91423	555-1234	
Jagielo, JoAnn	567 Main St.	Los Angeles	91423		
Jonson, Carol	567 Main St.	Los Angeles	91423	555-1234	
Lara, Alicia	567 Main St.	Los Angeles	91423	555-1234	555-1234
Lee, ViVi	567 Main St.	Los Angeles	91423	555-1234	555-1234
Levine, Rose			91423		
Lewis, Christine	567 Main St.	Los Angeles	91423	555-1234	
O'Brien, Bernadette	567 Main St.	Los Angeles	91423	555-1234	555-1234
Payne, Gail	567 Main St.	Los Angeles	91423	555-1234	
Pearce, Anne	567 Main St.	Los Angeles	91423	555-1234	
Pettit, Cheryl	567 Main St.	Los Angeles	91423		
Simmons, Ann	567 Main St.	Los Angeles	91423	555-1234	555-1234
Titurn, Caroline	567 Main St.	Los Angeles	91423		
Tomita, Lisa	567 Main St.	Los Angeles	91423		
Tucker, Christine	567 Main St.	Los Angeles	91423	555-1234	555-1234
Ulrickson, Jean	567 Main St.	Los Angeles	91423	555-1234	
Weatherly, Mary	567 Main St.	Los Angeles	91423		
Yearnshaw, Pat	567 Main St.	Los Angeles	91423	555-1234	
Young, Kathy	567 Main St.	Los Angeles	91423	555-1234	555-1234
Zentner, Lisa	567 Main St.	Los Angeles	91423	555-1234	555-1234

34 clients selected or 15.38% of your clients
Sex Female

Salon Transcripts
Client Selection

Name	Address	City	Zip	EvePhn	DayPhn
Agnos, Irene	567 Main St.	Los Angeles	91542		
Bagley, Elyse	567 Main St.	Los Angeles	91542	555-1234	555-1234
Baumann, Jerome	567 Main St.	Los Angeles	91423	555-1234	555-1234
Bell, Carol	567 Main St.	Los Angeles	91423	555-1234	555-1234
Bennett, Kathy	567 Main St.	Los Angeles	91423		
Biondi, Heather	567 Main St.	Los Angeles	91423	555-1234	555-1234
Cale, Toni	567 Main St.	Los Angeles	91423	555-1234	
Chun, Joyce	567 Main St.	Los Angeles	91423	555-1234	
Daley, Sue					
Dana, Deane	567 Main St.	Los Angeles	91542	555-1234	555-1234
Dudley, Brenda	567 Main St.	Los Angeles	91423	555-1234	555-1234
Genco, Jane	567 Main St.	Los Angeles	91542	555-1234	
Gosset, Loretta	567 Main St.	Los Angeles	91542		
Hafron, Andrea	567 Main St.	Los Angeles	91542	555-1234	
Hagen, Matthew	567 Main St.	Los Angeles	91542		
Handlen, Pam	567 Main St.	Los Angeles	91542		
Hartley, Jody	567 Main St.	Los Angeles	91423		
Hartman, Bob	567 Main St.	Los Angeles	91423	555-1234	555-1234
Ikesaki, Lori	567 Main St.	Los Angeles	91542	555-1234	
Jackson, Marian	567 Main St.	Los Angeles	91542	555-1234	
Kay, Ursula	567 Main St.	Los Angeles	91542	555-1234	555-1234
Knudsen, Carol	567 Main St.	Los Angeles	91542	555-1234	555-1234
LaPointe, Jeanne	567 Main St.	Los Angeles	91423		
Lewis, Christine	567 Main St.	Los Angeles	91542	555-1234	
MacBride, Robert	567 Main St.	Los Angeles	91542	555-1234	
Mancha, Vicki	567 Main St.	Los Angeles	91423		
Mathews, Kelly	567 Main St.	Los Angeles	91542	555-1234	
Nakamura, Joni	567 Main St.	Los Angeles	91542	555-1234	
Nootenboom, Michelle	567 Main St.	Los Angeles	91542	555-1234	
Orchard, Rebecca	567 Main St.	Los Angeles	91542	555-1234	
Pearce, Anne	567 Main St.	Los Angeles	91542	555-1234	
Pfiefer, Betty	567 Main St.	Los Angeles	91542	555-1234	555-1234
Ross, Shannon	567 Main St.	Los Angeles	91542	555-1234	
Titurn, Caroline	567 Main St.	Los Angeles	91423		
Tomita, Lisa	567 Main St.	Los Angeles	91542		
Tucker, Christine	567 Main St.	Los Angeles	91423	555-1234	555-1234
Vogel, Marlette	567 Main St.	Los Angeles	91423		
Ward, Rosalee	567 Main St.	Los Angeles	91542	555-1234	555-1234

38 clients selected or 17.19% of your clients.
Service Spending>100.00

Salon Transcripts
Client Selection

Name	Address	City	Zip	EvePhn	DayPhn
Agnos, Irene 4/5/97	567 Main St.	Los Angeles	91542		
Bagley, Elyse 4/18/97	567 Main St.	Los Angeles	91542	555-1234	555-1234
Balavage, Monica 1/6/97	567 Main St.	Los Angeles	91542	555-1234	555-1234
Curry, Ken 1/6/97	567 Main St.	Los Angeles	91542	555-1234	555-1234
Daley, Sue 4/18/97					
Fong, Curtis 1/10/97	567 Main St.	Los Angeles	91542	555-1234	555-1234
Genco, Jane 4/18/97	567 Main St.	Los Angeles	91542	555-1234	
Gosset, Loretta 4/14/97	567 Main St.	Los Angeles	91542		
Hafron, Andrea 4/18/97	567 Main St.	Los Angeles	91542	555-1234	
Handlen, Pam 4/14/97	567 Main St.	Los Angeles	91542		
Ikesaki, Lori 4/14/97	567 Main St.	Los Angeles	91542	555-1234	
Knudsen, Carol 4/5/97	567 Main St.	Los Angeles	91542	555-1234	555-1234
Lewis, Christine 4/5/97	567 Main St.	Los Angeles	91542	555-1234	
MacBride, Robert 3/17/97	567 Main St.	Los Angeles	91542	555-1234	
Mathews, Kelly 4/18/97	567 Main St.	Los Angeles	91542	555-1234	
Moeller, Alice 1/6/97	567 Main St.	Los Angeles	91542	555-1234	555-1234
Nakamura, Joni 4/18/97	567 Main St.	Los Angeles	91542	555-1234	
Nootenboom, Michelle 4/5/97	567 Main St.	Los Angeles	91542	555-1234	
Pfiefer, Betty 3/17/97	567 Main St.	Los Angeles	91542	555-1234	555-1234
Tomita, Lisa 4/14/97	567 Main St.	Los Angeles	91542		
Ward, Rosalee 4/14/97	567 Main St.	Los Angeles	91542	555-1234	555-1234
Young, Kathy 1/6/97	567 Main St.	Los Angeles	91542	555-1234	555-1234

22 clients selected or 9.95% of your clients.
Emp/Service Perm, emp:Sandra Smith after 1/1/97

FINDING THE RIGHT SYSTEM

When your salon is computerized, you are better equipped to meet the needs of clients. And, with care to your physical surroundings and in-house client handling methods, the added information derived from your computerized database will definitely help you meet your goal of owning a successful salon. To begin your search for the right system contact distributors and manufacturers whom you trust, to learn of software companies in the beauty industry. Read trade journals and do not hesitate to ask sales representatives for salon software referrals. If possible, attend trade shows and try their wares first-hand.

Always seek out a company's valued clients. Ask what positions they were in (technically speaking) when they began their program. Did they receive assistance? Does the software company offer regular updates for their programs? If your findings are not positive, keep shopping. Quality salon software companies are in a continuous state of development. These forward-moving companies can be your greatest allies in your effort to remain both current and prepared for future developments in our salon industry.

To begin your search for the right computer, contact distributors and manufacturers whom you trust, to learn of software companies in the beauty industry.

chapter 4

The Groundwork

1. Client records
2. Salon maintenance services
3. Salon supplies
4. Client surveys/questionnaires
5. Shopping smart

HOT*opic*

PERFECTING YOUR RECORDS

Compiling information and analyzing your situation is a great beginning to a more sophisticated care program. While you do not have enough information yet to create a contemporary client care program of your own, you can begin laying the foundation by perfecting your salon records. This process can take up to six months to complete and should never be hurried. Changes made slowly are much easier to accept, especially by your clients. Whenever possible, convey your new methods of doing business as *improvements* rather than changes, and share with everyone what the end result of a particular new action will be. This information will give your clients and staff positive anticipation of what is to come next. As for yourself, enjoy each step along the way as you modernize your client care program. Realize that as you proceed, each profile completed and every correct name inputted into your computer will make your salon a stronger, more viable business.

Gathering a Complete Profile

The basis for your client file is your client profile card. It is the only means to ensure that all your clients are in your computer with complete information. Before you can improve your record keeping in this area, however, you need to discover *why* they are incomplete. You will most likely find that many minor areas need correction. Your front desk, for instance, may not consistently ask for client profiles to be filled out, or your staff may not be concerned with the correct spelling of every client's name. Each problem area that is uncovered will not only give you the opportunity to correct the situation, but also will allow you to share positive information about what a good client database will create.

Communication is a great tool in diffusing most of the problems in this area. By sharing your new commitment to improved client record keeping with your entire staff before launching this portion of your project, you will have better cooperation and many quality suggestions for the best ways to accomplish this salon goal. And although you can not really share a "plan" that has not been formulated, you can express the salon's desire to improve client care and that the first step is to have a complete salon database. After all, with this information, the salon can offer selective promotions, celebrations, and special rewards for their loyal clientele. It is also the only way to romance the clients who have drifted away.

One suggestion to partially solve client misinformation is to have the front desk fill out all clients' names (first and last) on everyone's tickets before the start of each business day. This will also remind your salon coordinators of the importance of getting correct spellings when making all appointments, regardless of how long the client has been coming to your salon. The more difficult aspect of this delegation is to creatively re-budget their time to make sure this always happens. A separate meeting for your front desk staff would be most beneficial in ironing out the kinks in this area.

You should also consider implementing an electronic appointment book program in your salon. This particular function is a time saver because it automatically prints out the service tickets with complete information at the beginning of each work day.

Your Front Desk Team

It is extremely important that your salon coordinators understand the importance of this information and the effects bad records have on the salon's business. Together, you need to decide how to accomplish your goal of 100% complete records as it pertains to their interaction with the salon's clientele. The basics of having enough forms and clipboards for ease of filling out forms, and so on, should be organized. The time needed to get this information must also be integrated into their busy days.

Even more important, the objections that clients raise when asked to divulge personal information must be resolved. When you ask new clients for information, some may be hesitant to cooperate. After all, we are in an age where personal information, if released, can create anything from an avalanche of telemarketing calls to stolen identities. Assurances in this area are very important even when fears and objections are not openly voiced by your clients. Also, when a client has been in many times and you are belatedly asking them to fill

Consider implementing an electronic appointment book program in your salon.

out a profile card, diplomacy is also required. After all, you already know them, don't you? But, by providing a completed profile card, you can make their salon appointments more efficient as well as shower them with appreciation throughout the year.

Some valid reasons you may give clients for taking the time to fill out the needed information include not having to present identification for check writing in the future and being alerted of salon promotions, including coupons, gifts, and discounts. Your assurances to clients of complete information privacy should also be shared with your general staff as they will be diffusing many of the same objections.

Appointment Listings

One of the most difficult obstacles to overcome is taking the time to book each client properly. First and last names must be included in the appointment listing and they must be spelled correctly. If your salon is used to casual bookings, patience and perseverance will be needed. However, by establishing a system of checks, you can catch most of the problems no later than the day clients arrive for their appointments.

Client Information Checklist

- [ ] Check your books for client names versus your computer records on a daily basis for at least the first three months. Even if names come up correctly, look at profile information to make sure it is complete.
- [ ] Check your books versus your computer records intermittently thereafter (at least once a week).
- [ ] Check with your front desk to make sure they are receiving correct information from the stylists.
- [ ] Check with your stylists to make sure they are receiving correct information from your front desk.

Overcoming Attitude

Although you are changing things for the better, still expect a few sour faces in the beginning. Stylists do not like to disturb their clients by having them fill out forms, and the front desk often finds it difficult to get the needed data during their busy day, especially if it pertains to many names. But this phase will pass. Stay true to your vision of a top-notch database and very soon only your new clients will need to provide your salon with profile cards. The task will become smaller and proficiency will increase. In a relatively short period of time, life will once again become routine—a new routine that will help everyone in their quest to succeed.

> Stay true to your vision of a top-notch database and very soon only your new clients will need to provide your salon with profile cards.

Daily Book Checks

One effective step in updating your master client list is to have your front desk (or yourself) come in a few minutes early and run the names that are on your daily books through your computer. If they come up "unknown," highlight their names on the books with a bright pen and write "PC" (for profile card) beside them. Then have your staff ask these clients to fill out a profile card.

If a client comes up as "known," pull up the profile card and make sure it is filled out completely, including name, address, and telephone number. If it is not, have the front desk ask for their information when they show for their appointments. Once this activity becomes routine, it will take only a few minutes each day. You will be amazed at how much information you would have otherwise missed and how quickly your database will become 100% complete and accurate. If you are having someone else do your postings, this is also an excellent way to check the quality of their work.

Creating Time

Because you are asking your salon coordinators to spend more time on the salon's client records and their days may be already full, you must find ways to creatively rearrange their schedules to prevent additional payroll expenses. Consider the following:

- ✦ If you employ more than one salon coordinator, the solution is usually easy. Are there times during the day when their schedules overlap? Can you trim fifteen minutes off front desk time during this time period and allocate it to record keeping?
- ✦ Would your salon coordinators be willing to arrive fifteen minutes early and take an extra fifteen minutes for lunch? Since most front desk personnel "grab and run" their meals, the prospect of a longer lunch time may seem very attractive.
- ✦ Is your shop assistant available to help set up the front desk in the morning so that your salon coordinator is free to perform record keeping tasks?
- ✦ Can your evening salon coordinator set up the front desk for the next day as the evening winds down, to give the morning coordinator more time to accomplish the extra paperwork you now need?
- ✦ Can your evening salon coordinator participate in auditing your appointment books for names and information?
- ✦ Can your evening salon coordinator set up service tickets so that your morning coordinator has more time to check names and record cards?
- ✦ Can you personally allocate official time each day to do this?

However you ultimately decide to accomplish these extra tasks, always keep in mind that it is important to develop higher efficiency in all areas of your front desk so that you may accomplish these things without adding extra payroll expenses. And, always be aware that salon coordinators are like all other people who have established a routine in their job—added duties may seem impossible at first, but they are not. This crucial transition will go even more smoothly if you offer a choice of alternative schedules, brainstorm ways to become more efficient together, and always make them realize that they are an integral part of this program.

Positive changes are better achieved through inspiration rather than dictation. To encourage the growth of your salon in a more positive direction, business improvements should first come from you. Looking over your business evaluation, you will find many areas that you can begin improving while you are waiting for your client records to become complete. As the salon owner, ask yourself first, "What can I do to create an extraordinary experience for our clients?"

As the salon owner, ask yourself first, "What can I do to create an extraordinary experience for our clients?"

MAINTAINING A TOP-NOTCH SALON

One of the great ways you can immediately create a better experience for your people is to set a higher standard of physical salon care. How wonderful it is to walk into an establishment that has gleaming floors, sparkling clear windows, and freshly cleaned furniture! Your salon appearance is an important part of creating a pleasing environment and it is also necessary for your success. How you create and maintain this standard, however, will be determined by your financial state, as well as your own commitment of time and effort. What is your janitorial budget? Once you know this figure, you will know how much outside help you can afford to enlist in upgrading your situation. And unless your budget is abundant, be prepared to spend regular times throughout your week "loving your salon" through personal care.

Maintenance Services

Finding a good floor service you can trust and afford is a wonderful business discovery. Get bids from as many companies as possible before committing to one. Always ask for beauty salon referrals, and make sure the company you choose will give you a reduced price when their number of services/visits per month increases.

After you have established the price you will pay, carefully go over your budget once more to see how many times you can realistically afford floor services per month. Whatever the frequency, set up a regular maintenance schedule and between their visits, spot clean your salon often to help prolong the effect of their efforts.

With better client care your janitorial budget will naturally increase. Adding more frequent waxing and buffing services will further help the appearance of your salon. It will also motivate staff members to keep their areas in tune with the rest of their environment.

You should also evaluate your budget for other outside cleaning services. Consider a window service if your current floor maintenance company does not perform this job at a reasonable rate. Or, consider periodic cleaning of blinds and draperies. You may be fortunate enough to be able to afford a janitorial service that totally cares for your salon. If you do, your success in this area should be applauded.

If you are contemplating enlisting the aid of a janitorial service, interview the owner or manager carefully and put your expectations in writing.

If you are contemplating enlisting the aid of a janitorial service, interview the owner or manager carefully and put your expectations in writing. What is important to you? What details should *always* been done? What is the order of importance? Break down your cleaning "musts" per area and check them thoroughly after each visit.

Cleaning staff come and go frequently and after two or three people have joined and left a company, the people cleaning your salon may have no idea of your preferences. Always check their work against your expectations. If your goal is to significantly enhance your environment by paying for this service, make sure that you are satisfied. Also realize that having a complete service such as this is always a financial responsibility. It is your job to make sure it consistently makes your salon environment shine. Check and double check their work; do not hesitate to be picky. After all, don't your clients hold the highest expectations of your work?

Once you have determined your method of salon maintenance, it is important to put it in writing, making sure everyone knows what you are doing. Although better habits are sometimes hard to learn, your staff will be more willing to participate in future improvements if they see that you are taking the first step towards this goal. They will also learn to appreciate and recognize your efforts as these improvements continue to grow.

Tentative Guidelines of Responsibility

Things shared are often the most treasured. In Japan, students must clean their own schools and so, not wanting to create a mess for themselves, they have much tidier habits throughout the day. In fact, even though graffiti in Japan is still somewhat of a problem, the students traditionally write their scribbles in pencil.

So it should be with all members of your staff (this includes management). Many areas used by stylists such as their stations, the break room, and the lab need to be cleaned and maintained by them on a daily basis. Stylists also need to be aware of the permanent damage the products they use can do unless they are cleaned up quickly.

Management, on the other hand, needs to be responsible on a daily basis for other areas of the salon. The toughest part will be for everyone to consistently carry through on the responsibilities. So before you propose anything to your staff, think the situation through. Always be prepared to change your ideas, but never your standards, once they are up for general discussion.

For instance, does the salon management need to make sure that the rest rooms, retail and waiting areas are cleaned daily? Do all stylists clean their stations, mirrors, and floors nightly before leaving? Eventually, as your program unfolds, issues such as these need to be discussed then followed through to make sure they are not forgotten. The result will be a salon that is appreciated and treated with respect by all.

To maintain a pleasing environment, your salon will also need to establish hour-to-hour maintenance schedules for particular areas. Areas needing frequent checks are rest rooms, beverage areas, and the waiting room. While you may not have the support of a salon maid to help in these matters, you still need to devise a system that clearly spells out what needs frequent attention; then, make the commitment to follow through.

Improving your records and upgrading the physical condition of your salon can be accomplished without significantly involving your stylists. However, the effects experienced by you and your front desk as you institute your first changes will be profound. Work with your people and help them whenever possible. Always listen to what they have to say. Their input can make your future program a complete success or a dismal failure.

CLIENT SURVEYS

During this time period, you can actively involve your service staff by having them participate in creating and handing out your first client survey. Once finalized, you will have established a new standard for reaching your clients. The information you receive will open the eyes of everyone on your staff regarding their accomplishments and shortcomings, and will help everyone embrace the mindset that change is part of growing in business.

> Always be prepared to change your ideas, but never your standards, once they are up for general discussion.

A great blueprint for this activity has been produced by the Gary Manuel Salon of Seattle, Washington. They have a questionnaire that they send out to all new clients called, "Did We keep Our Promises?" As an incentive for clients to return it, they also include a coupon and offer a postage-paid method of reply (see figure 4-1a).

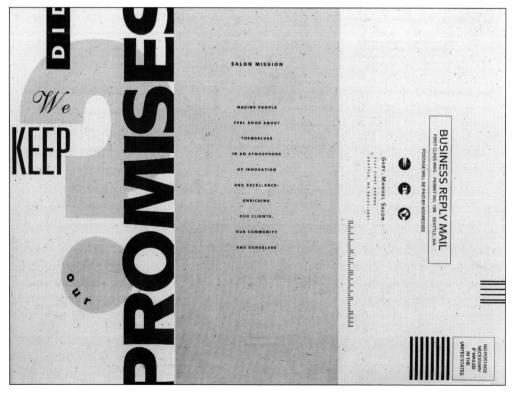

Figure 4-1a
Client survey for new clients. (Courtesy Gary Manuel Salon.)

"We also keep our surveys strategically placed around the salon," states co-owner Manuel Benevich, "and when clients are particularly moved about their experience that day, they can fill one out. We rarely get negative comments, but when we do, we telephone the person immediately. Our goal is to remedy the situation and have the client return to our salon."

When starting out, you might consider giving every client who visits your salon the opportunity to fill out a salon questionnaire, either by handing it out directly or mailing it to them shortly after their visit. To do the latter, of course, you will need to make sure your records concerning name and address are complete.

Allowing clients to tell you what they want, like, and dislike concerning your salon will give you the power to create a contemporary client service system that is accurately tailored to your business success. As in all relationships, communication will reveal some unexpected truths. Many of the things you may feel are most important to your clients could be secondary, and others which have been overlooked completely, may be critical to keeping them as clients in the future.

Creating Your Client Survey

It is important to keep the survey as brief as possible, while still receiving all the information you require for creating a better system. Creating such a questionnaire takes time and thought. Some things you should keep in mind when compiling your survey questions are:

✦ Whenever possible, ask an open-ended question (one that requires more than a "yes" or "no" reply).

✦ Multiple choice is also valuable especially when choosing such things as salon music. When doing this, always leave a space for "other."

✦ Try to word your questions so that you will receive constructive solutions. An example would be: "Please tell us ways we can improve our refreshments" instead of, "What is your opinion of our refreshments?"

✦ Leave space where clients may comment without being prompted. You may simply list this area as "other," or whatever you feel best encourages clients to communicate with you about things that are on their minds. Often, this special area will yield surprising results.

The Dead Spider Story

In a recent survey, a client confessed that despite great care by the salon, there was one detail that was absolutely driving him crazy. In fact, he confessed that he dreaded the shampoo service, because he knew "it" would always be there. "I've noticed the improvements you've made to the bathroom facilities and your stations," he wrote. "The shampoo area looks good, too. I only have one request. The dead spider that has been stuck in your light fixture over the third shampoo bowl for the last several months needs to be laid to rest. Can you help him?"

> Allowing clients to tell you what they want, like, and dislike concerning your salon will give you the power to create a contemporary client service system that is accurately tailored to your business success.

Dear Client:
Thank you for your recent visit to our salon. It is our goal here to meet the needs of all who visit us. To help us reach our goal, would you take a minute to answer the following questions. For being so kind to give us your information and time, bring in the top of this card and receive a 10% discount on your next services.

Thank you,
Bob Steele

1. Front Desk	Yes	No	Didn't Notice	Comments
(1) Was area clean?	☐	☐	☐	_____
(2) Were you treated well?	☐	☐	☐	_____
(3) Were services professional?	☐	☐	☐	_____
(4) Were your needs met?	☐	☐	☐	_____
(5) Staff who served you _____			☐	

2. Cleansing Area	Yes	No	Didn't Notice	Comments
(1) Did you get a good shampoo?	☐	☐	☐	_____
(2) Were you told what products were used on your hair?	☐	☐	☐	_____
(3) Was shampoo relaxing?	☐	☐	☐	_____
(5) Staff who served you _____			☐	

3. Hair Service	Yes	No	Didn't Notice	Comments
(1) Did your stylist listen?	☐	☐	☐	_____
(2) Were they running unreasonably late?	☐	☐	☐	_____
(3) Did they explain what products they used on you?	☐	☐	☐	_____
(4) Have you liked your hair?	☐	☐	☐	_____
(5) Staff who served you _____			☐	

4. Over all impression	Yes	No	Didn't Notice	Comments
(1) Was salon clean?	☐	☐	☐	_____
(2) Were we professional?	☐	☐	☐	_____
(3) Would you recommend us to a friend?	☐	☐	☐	_____

(4) What did you like the most? _____
What did you like the least? _____
What would you like to see different on your next visit? _____

Comments: _____
_____
_____
_____

☐ Bob: please keep my comments confidential
_____
Name (optional)

‖‖‖

NO POSTAGE
NECESSARY
IF MAILED
IN THE
UNITED STATES

BUSINESS REPLY MAIL
FIRST CLASS MAIL PERMIT NO. 16566

Confidential Reply to Bob Steele

Bob Steele
hairdressers
4355 Cobb Parkway
Atlanta, Georgia 30339

ıılılıllıııllııılılılılılılılıılılılılıl

Fold here second. Please tape, do not staple.

Tear here first.

Bob Steele
hairdressers
4355 Cobb Parkway
Atlanta, Georgia 30339
(770) 952-3556

Figure 4-1b
Client survey.
(Courtesy of Bob Steele hairdressers.)

While striving to improve the quality of your salon, it is very important that you view it from the same perspective that your clients do. You can do this most effectively by allowing room to express their opinions and concerns. Only then is the job truly complete!

Rewarding Your Clients

Offering a reward for completing the survey will entice many people to take the time to write down the requested information. For instance, purchasing a few cases of travel-size shampoo, and giving a bottle to each client who fills out the form will dramatically increase the response. If you are mailing the survey, send it return postage paid and include a coupon for their trouble (see figure 4-1b). This will not only allow you more success with your survey but will more than likely result in increased bookings.

The more anonymous the client is allowed to be, the more honest the answers will be. So include a preface that tells clients that you are intensely interested in what they have to say, but not equally as curious about who they are. They may, of course, volunteer that information on their own.

Voices from the Past

Past clients are less likely to reply, but those who do will give you some very good reasons why they no longer frequent your salon. Brace yourself for these responses and listen to what they have to say. Legitimate comments deserve everyone's concern and attention and so, as with all surveys, share the results with your staff. And, unless it is a personal complaint toward a specific individual, group discussions of criticism, applause, and suggestions are helpful. As a marketing suggestion for former clients, you might like to tag a coupon to your questionnaire that offers a free service (a haircut would be a strong gesture) with the stylist of their choice should they decide to return to your salon.

FUNDING YOUR PROGRAM

While the information in your records is slowly building, and your lines of communication are opening up, you can also evaluate your current expenses and discover ways to save significant amounts of money without compromising the quality of your services or supplies. It is amazing how much it costs to run even the smallest of salons and even more amazing to learn just how much money is being wasted by not shopping for the lowest prices, best perks, and products of comparable quality. The money saved from re-orienting your purchasing methods can help fund the improvements you want to institute without detracting from your paycheck, or your salon's overall financial stability.

Service Supplies

Service supplies can be dramatically discounted simply by shopping for good deals. Each month, many different deal sheets are sent to you from a variety of supply houses vying for your business. Start reading them! Begin giving greater importance to savings (as long as there is good phone service and a reasonable return policy), rather than to personal relationships you have with salespeople. The majority of our perks come from our product manufacturers and their exclusive distributors. You will not significantly reduce your opportunities for free education, specials, and personal promotions by shopping smart with your service suppliers. Perms, color inventory, and all the other service products we need to keep our doors open add up to a hefty bill at the end of the month. You can actually reduce your service supply costs by at least 20% when shopping *price* rather than *personality*.

You can actually reduce your service supply costs by at least 20% when shopping *price* rather than *personality*.

Service Supplies Check List

☐ Make a list of all major supplies you purchase including name brands, sizes, and average monthly consumption of each.

☐ Present this list to as many supply houses as you can find and ask them to bid prices on these products. Let them know that you are a busy, viable business that is interested in what they have to offer.

☐ Find out if they offer volume incentives by reducing the piece price when several of a single item are purchased.

☐ Volume discounts: How much do you have to purchase at any given time in order to receive a percentage discount on your overall purchase?

☐ If your supplies are being shipped, find out how much you have to buy in order to avoid shipping fees.

☐ Ask if they offer cash discounts when you pay c.o.d.

☐ Find out their criteria and policies on gifts with purchase. If you purchase twelve bottles of a single color tint, for instance, do you receive the thirteenth free?

☐ Do not hesitate to show them the amount of business you can generate for their company by sharing service supply receipts from recent months. If substantial, it will serve as a great incentive for them to give you the best possible deal.

☐ Audit your costs frequently. Service suppliers do not routinely alert you of price increases.

☐ Audit your sales tax charge on all delivery receipts. Are you being charged tax on items you legitimately resell? If you have not regularly done this in the past, do not hesitate to go back several months and double check your charges. It can add up to hundreds of dollars. You can deduct unjust sales tax charges on your next sales tax return, and stop further charges by providing a resell card to your supplier (confirm this procedure when ordering). If you do not do this, you could be paying up to 10% more for many of your products.

☐ Whenever possible, avoid service supplies that are only available through a single company.

☐ Begin comparing products, especially among such things as perm papers, pre-wrap lotions, cotton, rods, and clips. Cheaper products are often just as good. Always make sure to test market new products with your staff before discontinuing your current brands.

Shop Supplies

It is absolutely amazing how much disposable coffee cups, plates, toilet paper, and paper towels can cost at the end of the month. Although you cannot cease to supply these necessary items, you can cut down costs by being organized and shopping at wholesale houses. Not only do they sell facial tissue cheaper,

Audit your sales tax charge on all delivery receipts. Are you being charged tax on items you legitimately resell?

you can often purchase high-quality shop towels at incredibly low prices, and, you will find great tasting refreshments and cleansers for far less money than you would spend at the grocery store—even if you found them on sale.

By purchasing what you need in sufficient quantities to have a reserve, your clients will always have the products they need to be comfortable and content while visiting your salon. The only caution when shopping at wholesale houses is to make a list and stick to it. They are masters at offering you impulse items, mouthwatering treats, and many things in quantities you will never use.

And, of course, you will need to make sure that you have a safe, secure place for your purchases. Excess stock often leads to the "land of plenty" syndrome and a lot of waste can occur. Make a reasonable portion of supplies available and store the excess.

> The only caution when shopping at wholesale houses is to make a list and stick to it.

Shop Supplies Check List

- ☐ Never pay retail prices! Avoid grocery stores and convenience markets. Restrict your shopping to wholesale houses and discount department stores.

- ☐ Monitor your inventory. Leave out only what your salon needs to run comfortably. Lock the rest away and bring it out only as needed.

- ☐ Unless you own a very big salon, do the shopping yourself. Not only will you learn the best prices on items you use, but you also will learn new ways to save.

- ☐ Do not hesitate to purchase generic products. The money saved on generic counter cleaners, scrubs, laundry detergent, and so on is considerable and the slightly lower quality is barely noticeable even though the cost of savings are dramatic.

Bits of Waste

Finally, look for small things that might be causing big expenses. For instance:

- ✦ Do you have a water purification system or are you still buying expensive bottled water?
- ✦ Do you own a water cooler or are you still leasing one?
- ✦ Are you still paying for a laundry service or have you invested in a washer and dryer?
- ✦ Do you use bulk items whenever possible?
- ✦ Are you seeking wholesale outlets for your computer products?
- ✦ Are you using energy-smart light bulbs?
- ✦ Do you have control over your telephones, such as personal toll calls and even lengthy local calls?

You need to make your own checklist in this regard and, because every salon is different, you will discover many other things that can cumulatively save you thousands of dollars per year. The money saved will allow you to elevate the standards of your clients and staff, as well as yourself.

chapter 5

Outlining a Plan

1. Preparing the salon
2. By-products of service
3. The circle of care
4. Communication
5. Prebooking
6. Outlining a tentative plan

HOTopic

CREATING A PLAN WITH FLEXIBILITY

Once you have your records in order and you have taken some steps to improve the environment of your salon, you are ready to begin developing an outline for your contemporary client care program. This outline needs to be flexible because it only reflects *your* views and observations; it will serve as an invaluable guideline to begin discussions with your staff. Ultimately, it will help you vividly create the vision for your salon.

Before devising an outline, though, it is important to understand fully the concept of a contemporary client care program and how it can be molded to fit the needs of your business.

THE CIRCLE OF CARE

A contemporary client care program serves as a guide on how to offer your clients an extraordinary experience every time they visit your salon. It encompasses excellence in environment, service, and care, and also creates a continuous relationship with your staff. The "circle of care" is a major part of this program. It entails all aspects of the client's experience and will be the primary focus of your personnel.

Once clients become part of your program, they will receive great service, be thought about while away, and rewarded frequently for being part of your business. Your clients will soon learn that their patronage is appreciated.

Preparation Begins

Salon cleanliness is a major focus of client care and is accomplished in many different ways. New habits will need to be adopted by the front desk, stylists, and yourself. It will take time and patience to show people why cleanliness is important; following through with reminders will be necessary until everyone adopts cleaner, tidier habits. Having a cleaner salon will also take organization. How do you open in the morning to ensure that the salon is clean and fully prepared to do business? What happens during the day to ensure that it stays that way?

Preparation for salon visitors includes one hundred details compiled into a single message: "Welcome!" And as such, every aspect of your business that is thoughtfully prepared for the pleasure of your clients and staff are acts of professionalism that will be seen, felt, and enjoyed by everyone entering your salon. Think how important it is for all clients to be greeted by an environment filled with fresh air, having a tidy appearance, and offering refreshments. Also consider how nice it is to enter a restroom that is fresh and clean, or to be washed at a shampoo bowl that does not reek of stale chemicals left over from the frantic evening before.

The best way to prepare for the start of each business day is to begin preparations the evening before. Because staff members typically arrive at different times, and the ever present possibility of unexpected absenteeism, nightly preparation of work areas helps ensure that your salon is prepared to do business at the start of each day.

Figure 5-1
Stack your towels neatly as possible as opposed to leaving them bunched up and messy.

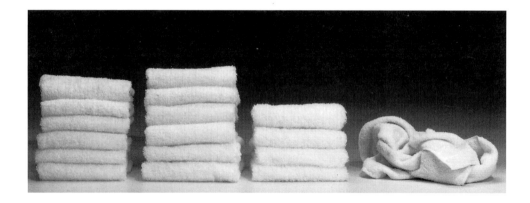

One dirty station in the midst of a sparkling shop will not only destroy the thoughtful efforts of everyone else, but speak miserably of the person who left the mess. Establish a routine where stylists clean up all chemical residue before departing each day. Leaving bowls of tints and bottles of solution for others to wash in the morning intensifies the reeking odors that seemingly multiply in a salon overnight. Also, always empty the trash before closing. The same applies to all parts of your salon. Evening tidying prevents morning clients from sitting next to stale coffee cups and cookie crumbs left from the night before and it sends an inviting and professional message to all passers-by who stroll by your windows at night. Magazines sloppily tossed about, used cups littering countertops and hair left on the floor after closing are eyesores to those who are on the outside looking in. Team effort between your stylists and the front desk will keep this problem well under control. But, again, be patient. Bad habits are hard to break and new ones, once acquired, will always need reinforcement.

Someone will need to be in charge of preparing the salon before opening. Sometimes called the "morning greeter," this person may be an assistant, salon coordinator, a designated stylist, or even yourself. It can also be several people who alternate taking on this role. The main thing is to make sure that the responsibility for morning salon preparation is clearly delegated and that you follow up periodically to ensure that it is being done up to the standards of your salon.

Your "morning greeter(s)" needs to make sure that:

- ✦ The salon is clean and tidy.
- ✦ Refreshments are ready.
- ✦ The salon smells fresh.
- ✦ The temperature is comfortable.

Scheduling staff is an art. As a business owner, it is important that all clients have a superb salon experience while at the same time salaries stay within budget. This can be done in many ways. When your staff cleans up after themselves, there is less time spent on set-up. By pre-counting and packaging your drawer the night before, you can simply place it in the cash register at the start of the next business day. And, by having the evening staff do some of the salon set-up as part of closing, your morning greeter will not have to come in quite so early.

Streamlining paperwork procedures are also cost-saving activities. In this regard, you have a wide range of possibilities. Because your paperwork system is unique to your salon, it will take some brainstorming with your front desk to come up with quicker systems.

When you first begin this portion of your program, people may believe that they need more time to accomplish a beautiful opening each day. Sometimes they are correct, but more often they simply need to get into a routine that is more efficient.

The best way to prepare for the start of each business day is to begin preparations the evening before.

Tips for a More Efficient System

Some general suggestions for creating a more efficient system are:

✦ Have your forms printed with as much information as possible so that your front desk does not have to take the time to hand write repetitive information.

✦ Have your service tickets and your client cards reflect the same order of information: name, date, service, retail, and so on, to avoid skipping and hunting while transferring information.

✦ Adopt a bar code system for your retail products to ensure a faster check-out.

✦ Never allow retail to be unpacked unless time has been allotted to code each product according to your salon system. Hunting for codes and manually looking up prices wastes time and prolongs client check-outs.

✦ Stock your front desk with everything it needs such as plenty of sharp pencils with eraser heads, pens, client profile cards, clip boards, and so on.

As you put your system into action, you will naturally experience some kinks for the first few weeks. But, as you and your staff learn to spend your time more wisely and act more responsibly as salon co-workers, debris will lessen and efficiency will increase to make this new standard a working reality—especially if you involve your staff, listen to them, and incorporate their ideas into making your salon open and close more professionally.

BY-PRODUCTS OF SERVICE

Many people working in our industry have become accustomed to hair on the floors, clipped nails scattered about, and used tint bowls foaming at their stations. The majority of our clients, on the other hand, have not. For example, how would you feel if you walked into a dentist's office and found teeth scattered all over the floor? This is an effective way to illustrate the impact we have on our own clients when we are messy. Loose teeth may not bother a dentist because he sees them everyday, but this same sight could haunt clients for months. It all depends on what you get used to.

Most clients find loose hair disgusting when it does not belong to them. Equally revolting can be messy clutter, someone else's dirty towels in their area, and any number of other things we handle on an hourly basis. Make your stylists aware of the effects by-products can have on their client.

The Toenail Story

There was once a very popular manicurist who always kept her area orderly and dusted. She was especially good with pedicures and did several of them each day. The staff of the salon loved her as a person and respected her work. However, staff members and clients shared the shampoo area where she tidied

> Many people working in our industry have become accustomed to hair on the floors, clipped nails scattered about, and used tint bowls foaming at their stations. The majority of our clients have not.

up her pedicure bath. The sink where she dumped her water several times a day was always filled with different shapes and colors of toenails. When it was brought to her attention by a staff member who was rapidly turning green, the manicurist could not understand what all the fuss was about. After all, she was knee deep in toenail clippings everyday and they did not bother her at all.

The moral of the story: Sensitivity to your environment and how others view your work is the first step to becoming more in tune with your salon's clientele.

A SINCERE WELCOME

Clients need to be greeted warmly when they arrive. Thinking of ways to make them feel special, acknowledging their presence immediately when they enter, and making them as comfortable as you would a guest in your own home are all part of a great experience.

Making sure that your salon coordinators are trained to greet each client with a smile, maintain eye contact, and call them by name, are all important points. It is also important to have good timing. Although it is not always possible to greet clients the moment they walk through the door, no one should be left standing in your reception area longer than thirty seconds without being recognized.

It is important to reassure each client by telling them that their service provider will be alerted of their presence. Then, rather than leaving a client wondering if his stylist is running on time, tell him approximately how long his wait will be before being serviced. A two-way communication system that keeps your front desk personnel from frantically running back and forth often works wonders in this regard.

It is also the responsibility of the front desk to alert other stylists when they are overwhelmed. Someone is almost always available to help. If the phones are frantic and people are not being greeted properly, pitching in until the crisis has passed is a beautiful gesture of team spirit. If this is something you would like to incorporate into your own plan, be sure to educate your staff on your front desk procedures.

One pleasing way to greet clients is to offer refreshments. They should be simple, tasty, and in tune with current consumer trends. Since caffeine is not always preferable, be sure to have herbal teas and decaf coffee available.

How you serve your refreshments will differ according to your philosophy. Your basic choices are Styrofoam, plastic, paper, or glass cups. Some argue that glass coffee cups are much better than their disposable counterparts, while others disagree; each has merits and drawbacks. Styrofoam and plastic are not

> Although it is not always possible to greet clients the moment they walk through the door, no one should be left standing in your reception area longer than sixty seconds without being recognized.

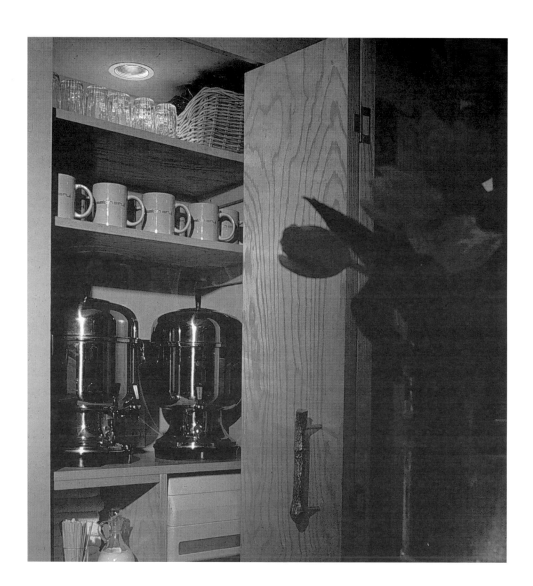

Figure 5-2
A clean, neat beverage area.

good for the environment in terms of volume of debris. Some believe that paper products waste trees. Many people feel that the texture of these materials are also unpleasant. Others simply feel that offering a beverage in a throw-away cup is tacky. Glass items certainly denote more quality but they are often not as sanitary as their disposable counterparts—washing dishes by hand in a salon environment is not usually equal to sanitary practices in a restaurant because chemical containers often are washed in the same sink. Unless your salon has a dishwasher (which is highly unlikely) the water will not be hot enough to sterilize the dishes. With the resistance to even antibacterial agents by many germs, glassware becomes a difficult issue. Additionally, glass cups require more counterspace.

The easiest answer would be to give your clients a choice. A simple sign can be put up by the refreshment counter, such as in figure 5-3.

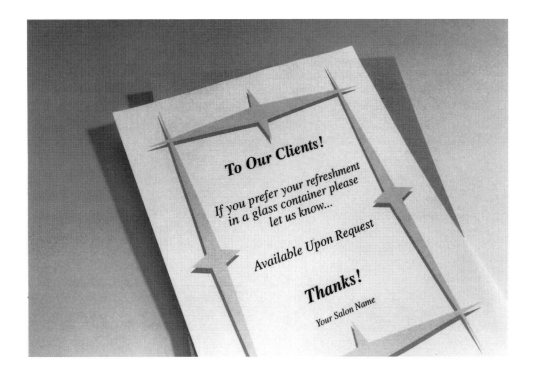

Figure 5-3
Refreshment sign.

Stylist Greetings

Greetings by stylists begin with cleaning their work areas. This means not only being ready for the *beginning* of the day, but all day. Remnants of previous clients' by-products should be removed before ever escorting current clients to their stations. Loose hair accumulated in the crevices of styling chairs, discarded towels, and so on all create negative impressions. Most clients will not comment on housekeeping if it is bad; they will simply fail to return to the salon. With an eye for detail and the willingness to take the extra minute to reorganize and clean, you will actually see a difference in your client retention. You also will be creating a healthier and more pleasant work environment for all fellow co-workers.

Walking to the front area and greeting clients before escorting them to the service area is also an important step in making all visitors feel welcome and at ease in your salon. Giving sincere eye contact, smiling, and addressing the client by name are things that communicate the very warm and reassuring message of "Welcome."

Planned Hospitality

By creating a greeting system filled with specifics, your clients will have a high quality experience each time they enter your salon. Professional greetings begin with the awareness that all clients should be treated as guests of your business whether it is their first or their one-hundredth visit. While it is important that every staff member share the spirit of this hospitality, it is equally important that they be given specific roles in the matter. If this is not made clear, positive intentions may turn into surprisingly negative results.

The Hello Story

A salon owner in Northern California decided that she wanted to improve the quality of her shop so she invested in a week-long seminar on salon business. The head lecturer emphasized how important it was to have all stylists share in the responsibility of making everyone's clients feel welcome. To help influence a change of behavior, this well-intentioned expert also talked at length regarding why everyone's business benefits from such an atmosphere.

The owner went back to her salon and shared information about the seminar, especially the part on greeting and caring for everyone's clients. At the end of her talk, the staff had a completely different idea of how they should act towards all customers of the shop. They readily agreed on the importance of smiling, giving eye contact, offering refreshments, and generally making all who came through the door as welcome as guests in their own home. The salon owner was very happy. The staff was delighted. It felt like a new beginning for everyone!

Three days later, an angry client greeted the working owner at her station after being processed through the front desk and shampooed by her assistant. When asked what was wrong, her client said, "I am really feeling uncomfortable here today. From the time I walked through the door until now, which hasn't been over ten minutes, I have been offered a cup of coffee five times by four different people, three different magazines and had to say 'hi' to every single person in the shop. What's going on?"

As always, good intentions are a wonderful beginning. But without a specific plan, goals are rarely reached. If the objective is to make sure that your salon atmosphere is both hospitable and professional, a system needs to be created that will achieve this aim in an organized, low-key manner.

Running on Time

Consideration of other people's time is also a driving factor in creating an experience that is positive and productive. While most of us are concerned about our own schedules and become agitated when clients are late, we often lose sight of the fact that when we are running behind, we could be affecting other peoples' lives as well.

Continuous care means taking your client at the appointed time. If your schedule is running late, contact that person to avoid undue inconvenience. It also entails responsibly booking people and resisting the temptation to work in un-

Continuous care means taking your client at the appointed time.

scheduled services when there is not ample room. Have the courage to turn away clients when they have pushed your schedule too far by arriving late. It also means that everyone on your staff show up for work on time and be focused on their clients the moment they walk through the door.

People feel relaxed, comfortable, and important when they are serviced promptly. They know that their own schedules are being respected and they can confidently work their hair services into their busy day. This attitude is contagious, spilling over into the salon and reinforcing the goal of an extraordinary experience for everyone.

PLEASURABLE CARE

Combined with a clean environment and an efficient booking system, pleasurable acts assail the senses of clients in every area of the salon. They begin with professional handling by the front desk and extend to the smells and tastes of attractive refreshments. Fresh smelling smocks, a warm greeting by their stylist, and a relaxing shampoo massage are all standard fare in a salon that practices contemporary client care.

Pleasurable acts also entail being sensitive to your client's needs. Striving to keep their backs dry and the water temperature exactly right while shampooing are just two small yet important parts of their salon visit. Also, there is simply a matter of quality.

- ✦ Do you have a consistent, prescribed routine while at the shampoo bowl?
- ✦ Do clients receive a head massage from a trained stylist or assistant?
- ✦ Are clients offered the right variety of shampoos and treatments for excellent results?

These considerations are key to servicing clients who want to remain with your business.

There is also the trend toward wellness in our society which should greatly affect how we provide service to our clients. People are looking for products and services that offer them a heightened sense of well-being and give them pleasure at the same time. For example, Adam Broderick Image Group in Stamford, Connecticut, puts relaxing drops of aromatherapy oils in their clients' palms just before shampooing. They are asked to rub their hands together, cup them over their nose and mouth, and breath deeply three times. Stylists always take the time to perform a massage ritual that has been taught to them by resident massage therapists. "We promise everyone a wonderful experience every time they visit us," Adam Broderick shares. "We always give the same quality massage on all clients, whether they've booked for a simple blow dry or a full day of services."

Noelle Spa for Beauty & Wellness in Ridgefield, Connecticut, continuously burns aromatherapy candles in their shampoo area. And what started out as a good head massage has now escalated to include the neck, shoulders, and arms. Co-owner Noel de Caprio comments, "Our clients loved their scalp massage so much that we just kept adding areas. With each one, the compliments became more frequent. We now move our chairs out, have the shampoo person stand behind the client and do a more thorough massage. It only takes five minutes, but the benefits have significantly contributed to our overall success." Their success has been astounding. Noelle Spa for Beauty & Wellness and Adam Broderick Image Group both employ over 120 people each and in excess of 15,000 square feet of working space. As they continue their growth, their focus remains on heightening the experience of their clients. To say that consistently providing special care for clients "works" is an understatement.

There are many other ways that we can add pleasure to our clients' visits. Smocks that feel good and look presentable help immensely with client comfort. Niceties such as cushioned shampoo bowls, comfortable styling chairs, and music that creates a better sense of balance are just a few other comforts you can provide to create pleasurable experiences during salon services.

Communication

In order to please people, we must also be able to communicate. Communication with clients by your staff can be accomplished through education and care. Surveys can do wonders for learning what is on the minds of everyone associated with your salon and feedback in the form of information, compliments, and promises do great things for people's confidence in your business.

You will need to decide if you want a formal consultation program or one that simply makes sure that key points are touched upon with each visit. Because salon professionals yearn to have as much independence as possible, you will want to balance what they need to do versus what makes them most comfortable. Again, joint discussions and agreements in this area are the best practice.

Points of Consultation

Some points you will want to consider covering are:

- ✦ Methods of making clients comfortable.
- ✦ Effective listening skills.
- ✦ How to pose open-ended questions.
- ✦ Ways to present professional products.
- ✦ Prebooking techniques.

Niceties such as cushioned shampoo bowls, comfortable styling chairs, and music that creates a better sense of balance are just a few comforts you can provide.

Excellent Services Through Advanced Education

There is also the challenge of consistently delivering excellent, innovative services. Providing advanced education and supporting an environment that promotes creativity are two important factors in your ultimate business success. While in years past educators in our industry have emphasized *business* education for stylists, it truly needs to be a 50/50 blend between business and technical artistry education. Without a growing knowledge of their artistry, clients will not be inspired by the services your salon provides.

Education requires large amounts of organization and goal setting. Besides holding regular classes in your salon and attending educational events in your area, it is crucial that your staff (and yourself, if you are a working stylist) receive regular hands-on training. To facilitate this, create an educational fund for your people. This fund can be set up in many different ways, all with the same result of higher education, excitement, and growth.

Gary Manuel Salon of Seattle, Washington, deducts $11.00 per paycheck from their employees. When the fund builds to between $7,000 and $10,000, their staff collectively decides what education they are going to buy with this money. Recently, their entire staff (including their salon coordinators) flew to Woodland Hills, California, and studied with Sebastian International for several days. Their fund paid for their hotel rooms and meals, as well as the educational event itself.

Diva Studio of Las Vegas, Nevada, does something entirely different but with similar results. They match their staff's retail commissions and when there is sufficient money in the fund, their salon stylists are encouraged to attend the workshop of their choice.

Regardless of the program you create, make sure your staff members are receiving extensive hands-on training at least twice a year and that the training they receive presents an artistic challenge to their current skills.

The message of contemporary salon artistry is "Be, grow, and create."

Michael Hemphill, owner of Michael Christopher Salon in Wilmington, Delaware, and NAHA Hairdresser of the Year in 1997, explains, "To attract the best clients, you need to have passion for your art. You should think, practice, and live your profession every day. Clients look for inspiration and guidance from us. If we deliver, they will remain with us for life."

Acts of Appreciation

There are also countless ways to tell clients how much we appreciate their loyalty. Verbal reinforcement is very important in any relationship. After all, how

> Besides holding regular classes in your salon and attending educational events in your area, it is crucial that you and your staff receive regular hands-on training.

do people feel when their significant other never says, "I love you"? What is the effect when a boss fails to praise a job well done? We need to hear, as well as feel, appreciation by those who are important in our lives. Knowing we are appreciated gives us the power to please, compliment, and reinforce our clients' acts of loyalty and support.

There are also more tangible ways to show how much we appreciate their business. These acts of appreciation come in the form of gifts, coupons, salon extras, and even sale privileges for those who spend generously at your salon. Add your own creative input into this category and the total suggestions and opportunities will be even greater. There are ways to thank all your customers, from the client who comes to your salon for the first time to the college student who visits twice a year. (Refer to Chapter 8, "Rewarding Your Clientele.")

The message of contemporary salon artistry is "Be, grow, and create."

PREBOOKING

This is an age-old problem. How do we get our clients to commit to prebooking? There are lots of ways, actually, and they become easier to accomplish once everyone realizes what it costs *not* to do so. If clients are due in six weeks and slip to eight because they do not think about an appointment until their hair needs attention, you will lose about two visits per customer per year. Multiply that times your entire clientele and the revenue lost is staggering. The solution? Prebook!

For example, if your salon has 2,000 clients, your average ticket is $30.00, and your salon does not prebook 50% of the time, you run the risk of losing $60,000 in gross income every year.

Another example: If a single stylist has 300 clients, an average ticket price of $30.00, and does not prebook 50% of the time, she will lose $9000.00 in gross income per year. If her commission is 50%, this is a direct loss of $4500.00 every year she works behind the chair.

Keep in mind that 50% is a very high average for prebooking. This percentage can run as low as 10%, creating losses of over $100,000 per year for salons and in excess of $8,000 a year in a stylist's paycheck. Start prebooking now!

Overcoming Prebooking Objections

Training your clients to prebook takes time and patience. It also requires technique and confidence on the part of those who are making the suggestion that clients prebook. But it can be done and the rewards for doing so are tremendous.

The most common response when a client is asked to prebook is, "I don't know my schedule. I'll have to call you later." When you think about it, how many

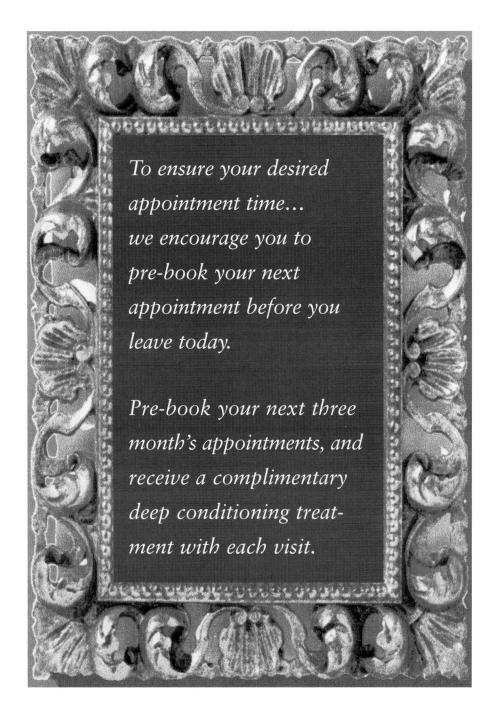

Figure 5-4
A pre-book sign.

To ensure your desired appointment time... we encourage you to pre-book your next appointment before you leave today.

Pre-book your next three month's appointments, and receive a complimentary deep conditioning treatment with each visit.

Figure 5-4
A pre-book sign.

of us really know what our schedule will be in five or six weeks? Yet, people prebook for doctor and dentist appointments all the time. The three most common reasons why clients resist prebooking salon services are:

1. They are not worried about getting in to see their stylist.
2. They have not fully accepted the fact that in order to look their best every day it is important to have appointments at regular, timely intervals.
3. They have no prior history of prebooking hair appointments.

Prebooking has not been an industry commitment since we abandoned the weekly set in the 1960s. This means that many baby-boomers and generation-xers have never prebooked a hair appointment in their life. Imagine that!

Failure to prebook not only costs thousands in lost service dollars, but retail sales suffer as well. When clients do not come to the salon at least every six weeks they will need to purchase new hair care products somewhere else. Most likely, they will refill their product inventory at a store closest to their home or work.

Prebooking is a key ingredient in being financially successful. But, it is much easier said than done. Clients naturally resist change. It takes patience and time for people to look at your business differently and take the extra step to commit to you as well as to themselves. However, there are things you can do to make prebooking a routine part of your services. It is a gradual process designed to re-educate your clients on how they look at you, your business, and their own beauty needs.

Prebooking is a gradual process so be patient and let things evolve naturally. Avoid the temptation to tell people you are full when you are not. Likewise, do not be intimidated when clients respond negatively because they can not get in to see you when they want to. They could leave you for another salon, but they probably will not. Either way, tending to your entire clientele is much more important than accommodating a client who has yet to realize the importance of your schedule. Part of your program is devising many other ways for prebooking to be accomplished. Brainstorming with your staff and working together will make it a reality for everyone in your salon.

Encouraging A New Commitment

Your clients will commit to their future services only if you make it personally important for them to do so. One of the best incentives clients have for prebooking is otherwise experiencing difficulty when trying to obtain an appointment on short notice. With excellent client care, your books will fill up naturally over a short period of time. As clients discover that they cannot get in to see you when it is convenient for them, they will begin making future appointments before leaving the salon—especially if a timely suggestion is made.

It is not uncommon for people to feel that their hair was left too long or that it grew out too fast between appointments. When these complaints are analyzed, something else will probably be brought to light: They have simply waited too long to return. Questions leading to a prebooking commitment include:

✦ How long has your hair been a problem for you?

✦ When were you in last?

✦ Was your hairstyle great for the first few weeks after your last appointment?

Failure to prebook not only costs thousands in lost service dollars, but retail sales suffer as well.

At the conclusion of each visit, asking the client how he liked his hair is a wonderful reinforcement for prebooking the next appointment. When your clients tell you they love what you have done, it is very natural and caring to reply, "I'm so glad you like it. Let's book your next appointment for x number of weeks and you'll continue to look great until we see each other again."

Your salon coordinators can be your most valuable team players in prebooking appointments. They woo, reassure and welcome everyone who sits in your chair. When the service is concluded, they should also suggest prebookings to all your clients. When this is done as a team effort, the results will be far more substantial.

Having stylists note when clients are due in for their next appointments (in weeks) on each service ticket is also a good way to help the front desk follow through with prebooking. However, the front desk should encourage prebooking only if the stylist has already verbally talked to their client. It is the role of the salon coordinator and the front desk to follow through with the prebooking, not to initiate it.

Following Through

Following through with the care of your clients is an act of professionalism that romances clients beyond the conclusion of their actual service. Some examples of follow-through are:

- ✦ Providing written literature on how to care for their hair, skin, and nails with specialized literature for care after perms, color work, and other chemical services.

- ✦ Calling clients to remind them of their appointments. This eliminates the majority of no-shows and also demonstrates extreme professionalism. There is also a substantial savings in terms of replacing clients on the books with others who want a quicker appointment.

- ✦ Calling all chemical service clients within three days of receiving the service to ensure that they are happy and working well with their hair. This adds to client retention and, if at all possible, should be part of your program. (The majority of your follow-up calls will no doubt be positive. The primary purpose of this function is not to weed out negative situations but rather |to create an even more positive experience by offering extended care beyond the salon visit—a unique experience for most clients!)

- ✦ Creating a formal waiting list. Clients appreciate this service and your staff is much happier knowing that the front desk is dedicated to helping them maintain a full book.

- ✦ Calling or sending out surveys to all new clients. Also, survey all your clientele at least once a year. (Refer to the Gary Manuel survey, "Did We Keep Our Promises?")

Having stylists note when clients are due in for their next appointments (in weeks) on each service ticket is also a good way to help the front desk follow through with prebooking.

- Following through with thank yous and gifts for everyone who refers clients to you. This is a great gesture of goodwill. Referrals go a long way in creating deeper bonds with your salon and also encourage clients to continue sending new people your way.
- Instituting "Acts of Remembrance." Birthday cards and gift certificates are always nice gestures. When you are computerized, you can even celebrate the date your best clients first came to your business. And, of course, there are always the holidays to remember your clients.

The Completed Circle

When your client arrives for a prebooked appointment, your circle of care is complete. By continuing the same efforts you previously made to arrive at this point, she will continue to return, along with her family and friends. Good service means great retention, plenty of referrals, and a solid chance to achieve the dreams you have for your own personal success.

A TENTATIVE OUTLINE

After sorting through all this information and adding categories that are important to your particular business, you are finally ready to devise a tentative outline of your contemporary client care program. Once completed, you can present this information to your staff and after discussions, a more concrete and detailed plan can be achieved. Be prepared, however, to change parts of your program for many months to come and, at least once a year, be prepared to review your entire client care program to ensure that it is effective and up-to-date.

Setting Salon Goals

As you begin your first written outline, take the time to set some tentative goals. In regards to financial matters, have your accountant "crunch some numbers" to validate your goals. Then consider the following:

- Review your growth thus far.
- Go over all your business reports once more.
- Check and double-check the walk-through you performed on your salon.
- How is the mood in your salon?
- Are things running better already?
- What results have you received from your surveys?
- What changes do you still need to make?

What do you want to accomplish through your new program?

- Better client handling? If so, how?
- More profit? What percentage? What dollar amount?

- ✦ A larger client database? If so, how big?
- ✦ Business security? In what way?
- ✦ Less time in the salon? How much less?
- ✦ More quality time in the salon? How much?
- ✦ Harmony? Describe it.
- ✦ Better staff retention? How will it be measured?

Answers to these questions will supplement your first client care goals with wisdom and a bit of history that you have already managed to accumulate. Write down your answers as vivid goals—be very specific. Using words such as "big," "a lot," "more," or "less" are too vague. When writing your goals, do not rush. You are planning your business success in real terms and that takes time, a lot of soul searching, and even some relaxation to allow your mind to wander through all the possibilities.

Creating The Outline

When you begin formulating the plan, it is important to gather information from as many people as possible. You are the first person to put together views and ideas; later, solicit information from your management team, salon coordinators, and stylists. In the end, your salon will not only have a more comprehensive client care program, it will also be the creation of everyone who is involved in making it a success.

Keep in mind that, even after your plan is firm, it will be a very long time before all your listed steps become a working reality. In the beginning, the magnitude of your proposed changes may seem more like a fairy tale than the future of your salon. But it will eventually happen if you make your plan one that reflects the mutual ambitions of the sterling members of your salon. After you have completed your first contemporary client care outline, you have reached the point where you can involve your management team and staff. Congratulations!

Creating a Step-by-Step Plan
Envision each step as a separate project for your business.

Cleanliness—By now, you have walked through your salon at all times of the day and evening and you have a good idea of the image your salon is projecting to those who come to you for services. Now:

- ✦ Set standards for a complete maintenance plan.
- ✦ Review your maintenance plan once more.
- ✦ Specifically delegate responsibilities for maintaining order during the day, including:

Reception/waiting area

Retail shelves/area

Service areas

Bathrooms

Lab

Breakroom

Other

✦ Schedule when and how you will always follow through with clients.

Welcome—This is your opportunity to provide a system that always starts every client visit on an extremely positive note.

✦ List what needs to be done in order for your salon to be fully prepared to open each morning.

✦ List cleaning procedures for the evening. Delegate responsibility.

✦ List cleaning procedures for the morning. Delegate responsibility.

✦ Write down ideas on how to streamline your system so it can be more cost effective.

✦ Establish criteria for your refreshment area. Are you going to offer glass, disposable, or both types of cups? Also, make a list of contemporary refreshments to be offered.

Greetings—Knowing the influence of your first hello to each client, make a list of what you would like to see happen every time a client comes in contact with your salon. Include:

✦ Telephone greetings.

✦ Greetings by your front desk.

✦ Greetings by your stylists.

Running on time—Knowing that running on time means retaining business, think about ways this can be accomplished effectively nearly all the time. Include:

✦ A policy on promptness.

✦ A policy on integrity of appointments.

✦ Time parameters for booking by the front desk.

✦ Teamwork ideas to help everyone keep their promise of promptness.

Pleasurable acts—Think of as many ways as you possibly can to heighten feeling of pleasure and well-being for every client who receives services at your salon.

✦ Use your five senses.

- List each area that your clients come in contact with in your salon. Make improvement suggestions for:

    Waiting area

    Front desk

    Retail shelves/area

    Rest rooms

    Changing area

    Shampoo area

    Service areas

    Exit

    Other

Communication—Communication is the major key to service satisfaction and a fully developed salon experience.

- Research and list classes you can attend that promote communication. Do not forget major hands-on workshops in this area.
- Enroll in classes that teach communication skills.
- Read books that cover this subject.
- List ways you already know how to:

    Compliment and encourage clients.

    Listen more effectively.

    Talk more sensitively.

    Express thoughts more clearly.

- List points you feel must be covered in every consultation.
- Set standards for consultations.
- Establish ways to tangibly say "thank you."

Excellence in services—Inspired stylists produce inspirational styles, excitement, and ongoing interest for their clients.

- List ways to increase education. Consider retail incentives, performance accomplishments, and cooperative funding.
- List types of education you desire, such as:

    academy training

    workshops

    guest artists

    trade shows

    staff

    other

- List frequency of attending educational classes, workshops, or shows.
- Create incentives for maintaining a high frequency of education.

Acts of appreciation—While communicating often encompasses verbal thank yous, there are also many other ways to tell clients that we appreciate their business. (This area is covered in detail in Chapter 9. For now, however, create your own ideas on ways you would like to thank and please your clients.)

- Give coupons. How many ways can you give your clients gifts through coupons?
- Give special considerations. What rewards can you envision bestowing upon your clients who fall in the top 20% of your database?
- List other ways to make all clients feel special.

Prebooking—Work to stabilize your business by creating a predictable pattern of earnings. Prebooking generates thousands of dollars annually, even for the smallest salons. Work on ways to:

- Overcome objections to prebooking.
- Receive a commitment from staff as well as clients to prebook.

Follow-Through—By extending care to your clients after their service has been completed, you will have demonstrated a high standard of professionalism.

- Establish a "reminder call" system.
- Establish a follow-up procedure for chemical services.
- Jot down ideas on how to create a formal waiting list.
- Consider sending thank yous and gifts. How many ways can you think of to thank and bestow gifts upon your clients?
- Consider Acts of Remembrance. Make a specific list of times when this is appropriate.

Enactment
of Change

chapter 6

1. Involving your staff in change
2. Unveiling the circle of care
3. Working through issues of change

HOT*opic* 4. Surveying your staff

CONFERRING WITH YOUR STAFF

Now that you have taken the time to analyze and create ways to upgrade your salon, you are ready to begin listening to what others in your organization have to say. If you have a management team, they should be the next group of people you confer with. Otherwise, a meeting with your entire staff is your next logical step, followed closely by a meeting exclusively with your front desk personnel.

Once you have completed your initial findings, your paperwork can be impressive in size as well as content. Because you want to hear what others see and think, you should set aside the majority of your own findings for a moment and allow your staff to make suggestions on ways to improve the salon. Share a bare outline of your circle of care in your first meeting and encourage them to fill in their own ideas and suggestions. You can then add your own thoughts and discuss everything.

A great awareness exercise you can do with your staff is to simply have them list at least five experiences where they have personally received great client care and at least five others where their care was poor. Each instance can be discussed, including as many details as possible. Be sure to have each person include the outcome of their experience. Did they remain and refer others or leave? Also ask them to share their feelings concerning what they look for in a business before becoming a loyal customer (this could be a clothing shop, restaurant, or anything that interests them). Is it attitude? Hours? Merchandise? Quality?

Defining the Program

In order for your staff to become involved in your program, however, they must first understand what great client care really is and why it holds the opportunity for them to become more successful in their own careers. Sharing the concept of the circle of care is an excellent means of defining exquisite treatment. A record of their performance to date is also powerful information and a great inducement to improve their situation. This can include current salon retention figures, prebooking percentages, and all other pertinent information that reflects their current success rate. And there is always the simple question, "Does your career provide you with the lifestyle you had hoped for when first entering this business? If not, why not?"

Defining the Program of Care

The circle of care covers all areas where clients are in direct contact with the salon. As such, they are also of prime importance to everyone on your staff. The contemporary client care program involves the circle of care as well as many other things that make the entire program a success.

Taking the time to prepare your material, organize your agenda, and listen to other care alternatives your staff may feel are important are all part of having this vital first introduction be a success. Because it is specific to your business, it must be created by you. Some of the points you should consider covering include:

- ✦ An honest discussion about what your staff likes most and least about their careers.
- ✦ Do they have vivid career goals? What are they?
- ✦ Ask your people to voice their feelings on how motivating a consistently full set of books would be. Solicit specific information. Are they always busy now?
- ✦ Discover how important a stable income is to their lives. Do they already have one with little fluctuation?
- ✦ Client retention figures of stylists (given individually for analysis during the discussion, but not openly shared with the group).
- ✦ Client retention figures for the salon as a whole.
- ✦ Prebooking figures by stylist (not openly shared).
- ✦ Prebooking figures for the salon.
- ✦ The power of prebooking. Share specific results.
- ✦ A breakdown of services by stylist (not openly shared).
- ✦ A breakdown of current services offered at the salon.
- ✦ Share a successful mix of services and what it means to income.

- ✦ Review paperwork and include anything else you feel would motivate your staff to raise their own standards of care.
- ✦ An overview of the circle of care: WHAT it is, WHY it is being used as a guideline for better care, and HOW they have control over its content so that it can fit comfortably into their lives. Emphasize what benefits them directly, as well as the total salon.

Do not expect to complete your circle of care discussion in a single meeting. It will require a series of meetings, possibly lasting months. Plan on spoon-feeding information to your staff and receiving input from them; also avoid tackling a new step before the previous one has been mastered. Above all, make sure your staff has made the commitment to improve client care before implementing any part of your plan. This will gradually reshape and tailor your program to be much more meaningful in the long run.

Allot plenty of time when you meet to review, reinforce, and congratulate everyone on their efforts to date. It will give your staff peace of mind and the chance you need to make your program a success. The old adage, "Rome wasn't built in a day" takes on a more vivid meaning when you apply it to your own salon—patience will be a big part of everyone's success.

To utilize time more wisely, consider talking about some subjects in-depth and others in more general terms, saving some for a later date when the bare necessities of your program have been perfected. Do not expect your staff to have the same focus as you must have in order to succeed. Management sees the big picture and all the details. Your staff, on the other hand, needs to have a clear understanding of the big picture and all the details that pertain to them.

STAFF MEETINGS

Salon meetings are the lifeline of salons. The key is to establish regular meeting times and remain faithful to them throughout the year. As with all challenges of owning and managing a salon, creating a successful meeting system can take time and patience.

Meeting formats can vary. The one thing all meetings should have in common, however, is a positive tone. Complaint sessions encourage discontent and helplessness. Addressing problems in a constructive manner, on the other hand, allows everyone to realize they have the power to improve their work environment as well as guide their own careers toward success.

Margo Blue Salon and Day Spa, in Charleston, North Carolina, for instance, does not allow complaints to be brought up unless staff members are willing to make positive suggestions to remedy the situation. It makes a big difference in the mindset of the staff and allows them more freedom to openly discuss

> Salon meetings are the lifeline of salons. The key is to establish regular meeting times and remain faithful to them throughout the year.

problems. Michael Christopher Salon, on the other hand, invites staff members to write down their complaints and put them in a hat. During the course of their meetings, a member pulls one complaint out of the hat, reads it aloud, and invites discussion and solutions. As the owner, it is up to you to first share your policy on this issue and then guide your group toward positive, proactive behavior at all times. If you do this, your staff will soon learn to focus on solutions themselves.

Some salons, such as Gary Manuel, prefer to have volunteer staff members form committees on certain subjects and then bring their findings back to the entire salon. This method helps the group focus on important topics through the guidance of their peers. It can also speed the process. The important key is to have staff members who are willing to donate their time. If you do not have such resources in the beginning, you may have later as things progress and people realize they can be an important part of the planning process.

The regularity of your staff meetings will vary according to the needs of your salon. Many salons meet monthly while others prefer a once-a-week or even twice-a-month schedule. During particularly heavy planning times, such as when developing a client care program, frequent meetings might be necessary and once established, monthly meetings could suffice. You might also consider planning for hectic times by readjusting your meeting schedule each year. You could plan a more comprehensive meeting the last part of November, for instance, and then not meet again until after the New Year when things resume a more normal pace. Whatever you decide, it is best to book these meetings out several months in advance so that everyone can mark their books accordingly.

The meeting time will also greatly depend on your normal salon schedule. Evening meetings are best for some salons while others find them difficult. Other salons plan their meetings in the morning before services begin. This, too, has its pros and cons. You should poll your staff, evaluate your salon schedule, and then pick the time that suits the majority of your people.

It is equally important to make all your meeting informative, uplifting, and productive. This requires a great deal of planning on your part to ensure that the goals of your business are met during these times and that the meetings themselves are the primary motivation for 100% attendance by your staff. Meetings that belabor subjects, even extremely interesting ones, become dull. One of the best plans is a one-hour meeting broken down into four separate fifteen-minute segments. This is particularly effective after planning sessions for your contemporary client program begin winding down.

1. Fifteen minutes of news and routine business announcements.
2. Fifteen minutes of hard skills (technical) education.

3. Fifteen minutes of soft skills (non-technical) education.

4. Fifteen minutes of fashion and style discussion/presentation.

This plan informs staff members of all events in the salon. It also gives everyone an opportunity to share techniques and new products and enables stylists to continue improving communication skills, business techniques, and so on. The style and fashion segment keeps both management and stylists abreast of the designers and trends that ultimately inspire all beauty creations.

Spicing your roster each year with periodic guest speakers will also enliven your meetings. To keep meetings fresh and lively, consider bringing in an educator/ motivational speaker at least once a month. As with all things, book your guest speakers in advance and confirm the booking at least one month before they are scheduled to appear. Look to your manufacturers for help. They often have hands-on classes that can be performed in a short amount of time, though you should make sure that what they will be teaching is appropriate to the skill levels of your salon. Also, network within your own clientele. Psychologists, chiropractors, accountants, and even personal shoppers are usually happy to share their expertise for either free or modest service trades. Businesses such as trendy clothing shops, modeling schools, and even nutritional counseling centers are often glad to share their expertise with a willing crowd. Remember that you and your staff have tremendous power when it comes to sharing news with an attractive target market. Position your business as a prime source for referrals and you will be amazed at the free education your salon will receive.

> To keep meetings fresh and lively, consider bringing in an educator/ motivational speaker at least once a month.

Having a full staff at all meetings can, in many ways, be your greatest challenge. Including all staff members in all phases of your meeting planning will greatly help. The content to be covered, the time allowed for each meeting, and the frequency of those meetings should be agreed upon by the majority of your staff. Once this is accomplished, it is up to you to make sure that everyone respects the schedule. It is also important to remember that your commitment to staff meetings comes in the form of planning and presenting consistently good material. Your staff should show their commitment to the salon by attending these meetings.

As you progress, you will find that many staff members will show up faithfully while others will challenge your new system. Not showing up for meetings and booking clients during these times are two common problems. It is important to remain firm. Staff meetings need to be a condition of employment. When hiring people, this policy should be firmly agreed upon before accepting anyone as an employee of your salon. You need to continually educate your veteran members on the importance of succeeding together and staff meetings are a vital part of this goal.

8 POINTS OF THE CIRCLE OF CARE

As tentatively outlined in Chapter 5, your contemporary client care program includes the following 8 points:

1. Cleanliness
2. Welcome
3. Running on time
4. Pleasurable acts
5. Communication
6. Excellent services
7. Prebooking
8. Follow-through

1. Cleanliness

This topic can be addressed any time after giving the overview of your program. When you do, be sure to share the efforts you have put forth to date. Give every staff member an opportunity to view your maintenance schedule and then post it in an area that is highly visible to your staff. Allow them to express their views on your commitment to salon maintenance. Do they recognize your efforts?

You can also share your commitment on improving hourly upkeep of the salon and explain what you have already done in this area. Listen to your staff, and let them share the problems they encounter due to unkempt conditions. Ask their opinion of what they feel is your responsibility as manager and what they are responsible for as staff members. This type of discussion establishes the

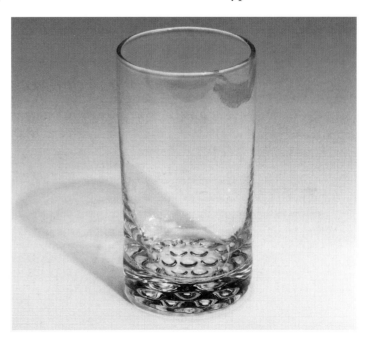

Figure 6-1
A dirty glass.

baseline for what you need to do to pull your people together and work as a team—yourself included! Are you hearing words of responsibility, or is the tone one of blame? Do they feel they should maintain their own work areas all the time? Do they do this?

Stylists who only clean up when they are not busy put many things in jeopardy: the client in their chair, their clients who follow that appointment, the clients of those around them, and all the clients of the salon who enter an unprofessional environment that is immersed in visual chaos. When stylists think only of the client in their chair and not of all the clients in the salon, they jeopardize business. Like a forest, watering only a single tree will cause the entire forest to die. But if they care for the forest, all the trees that make up this beautiful landscape will live long, fruitful lives. Superb care means providing good service for the person in your chair, those around you, and all the clients who will follow that day.

Where does your staff's responsibility begin and end? In the service areas only? What about the lab and break room? These are important issues you will need to work through. To do this, begin the process of establishing firm standards of responsibility, expectations, and performance. One of the most productive things you can do is enlist the aid of your staff in establishing a cleanliness standard for the salon. Some salons utilize their entire staff to initiate and complete this process while others, especially those with larger staffs, have a peer committee work on the standards first, bringing their results to the entire group to discuss and refine. In the end, put your finished product in writing, have it printed, and distribute it to everyone working in your salon. It is also a good idea to post it in places that are in plain view of your staff throughout the day.

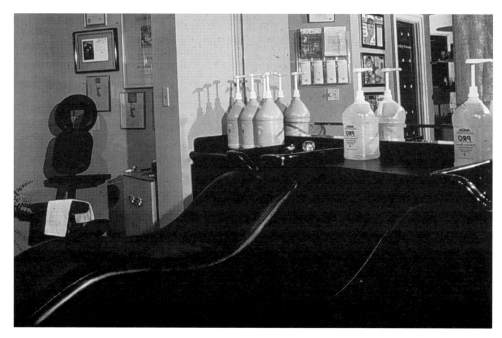

Figure 6-1a
A clean shampoo area.

How a clean and tidy shop is maintained will also need to be resolved. You have your schedules worked out and you have also established how to check your salon regularly during the day. Now it is your staff's turn to look at the total salon environment and make suggestions on what needs to be cleaned in the salon and how it can best be achieved.

Remember the walk-through outline you prepared when you first analyzed your salon? You will need it again. This time, though, your walk-through will be seen by many eyes instead of just yours. Your staff should have their turn at checking the salon and comparing all the areas against their five senses. It will help them look more sharply at their role in it's appearance, and at what needs to be accomplished by management to make the environment superb. Ask them to make suggestions on ways to improve any areas that are not up to par, and to compliment those that are. You will receive many great ideas this way and the process will empower your staff with the knowledge that they, too, have the opportunity to create change.

As a suggestion, you might want to have them walk through the salon in the morning before it is cleaned. Evening walk-throughs lack the strong impact of a morning check because your staff members have been immersed in the environment for many hours before the meeting. Clients enter the salon from a fresher perspective, making all their senses perceive the situation more sharply.

Part of the education of this walk-through is to upgrade not only the physical condition of the salon but also to become more sensitive to how clients see your business. Be sure to have your staff walk through with the mindset of "customer" as well as salon professional. The simple exercise mentioned earlier in this chapter about sharing other types of businesses where they are customers, what they have seen (good and bad), and so forth, is usually a great preliminary talk prior to a salon walk-through. Reviewing client surveys regarding their physical observations of your salon also helps sharpen the senses.

Staff walk-throughs are particularly valuable because there are many eyes making observations on ways to improve the total salon and staff members are privy to a lot of client complaints that are usually not shared with management. You will likely discover many things you have overlooked and will learn countless new ways to improve your business. Consider conducting a staff walk-through about every three months. It will keep your improvements on the mark, and help everyone remember the importance of a beautiful environment.

When you first begin your walk-through, be sure to take the same path as your clients—through the front door. Have everyone stand outside for a few minutes and encourage them to take a few deep breaths of fresh air. This will help make their first encounter with the salon environment closer to what their clients experience.

In the end, put your finished product in writing, have it printed, and distribute it to everyone working in your salon.

Allow the group to go over each area and situation separately. Even though some of the information may seem redundant, there is a message that is being learned and accepted: Cleanliness is a key component to client retention and prosperity; without it, everyone's success is jeopardized. Make sure that your staff realize the power they have over their careers by embracing a new standard of excellence in their deeds and actions throughout the salon. When this discussion is concluded and your staff has helped set the standards for their own cleanliness, produce a written procedure that lets them know what is acceptable in their salon and what is not.

Gross Encounters of the Third Kind

Have you ever been in a restaurant and found dried egg on your fork or a lipstick print on your glass? Have you ever laid down in a tanning bed that was soaked in the sweat from the person before you? Does just thinking about these things make you cringe?

Think about the wads of hair that may be in your own sink traps and imagine what your clients are feeling as they are asked to lay their heads back into a repulsive pile of loose hair. Imagine how clients feel when they are seated in a chair that still has the remnants of previous haircuts. What are they feeling when bowls of tint from previous clients are left on your counters, along with towels and tools, making it impossible for them to feel safe and comfortable while receiving their services.

Assuming the client's point-of-view is the best teacher of better habits.

2. Welcome

This important issue initially needs to be discussed by everyone. Offering compliments and suggestions by all members of your staff is the best way to begin establishing an excellent client greeting system. Your salon coordinators can also share their front desk experiences with the staff and the staff can do likewise. Hopefully, much of what will be shared will be positive. By also vocalizing complaints in a group situation, everyone can pitch in and begin offering solutions to improve things. Do not allow this to become a complaint session! Make a firm rule that solutions must always be part of any complaint brought up by the group.

> Make a firm rule that solutions must always be part of any complaint brought up by the group.

Keep in mind that you will be having a separate, thorough meeting exclusively with your front desk. The information that you glean from your general staff meetings will give you at least a partial basis to begin improving your front desk system.

For the entire staff, however, the first step to creating a wonderful welcome for your clients is to make sure that everyone in your salon acts as a team member. Part of that teamwork involves mutual consideration for the client, front desk, and stylists. Some of the points that your entire staff can work together on are:

- Firmly defining everyone's responsibility in greeting clients and making them feel welcome in the salon.
- Keeping the front desk informed when a stylist is experiencing scheduling difficulties.
- Standardizing booking procedures for the salon. If stylists work differently than the salon norm, these booking preferences should be put in writing and given to the salon coordinator. They, in turn, need to be organized so that they can be referenced easily when booking appointments.
- Instituting a policy of no loitering at the front desk. It makes clients feel uncomfortable, looks extremely unprofessional, and detracts from the attention all clients deserve.
- Channeling front desk complaints (by either clients or staff) through management. This is especially true of chronic problems. Frequent complaints between stylists and front desk personnel can create hostilities, causing client care to suffer from this unnecessary friction.
- If permitted, available stylists can lend a helping hand with the front desk when it is momentarily swamped and unable to offer exemplary care to those waiting for services. If stylists are not trained in desk procedures, they can still extend their assistance by helping clients with forms, offering refreshments, and notifying stylists that their appointments have arrived.
- Greeting each client warmly with a genuine smile and good eye contact are things that all clients should experience.
- Verbal greetings that make clients feel extremely welcome are also part of a beautiful salon experience: "Hello, Mrs. Jones, it is so good to see you. How have you been?"

Walking up to clients and warmly greeting them before a service is a very reassuring act that sets a positive tone. A brief touch on the arm, a handshake, or a reassuring pat are all part of the unspoken language we communicate with our people: "Glad to see you. You're going to receive a wonderful service."

Deciding as a group how to approach, greet, and escort a client back to the service area are key points that cannot be taken for granted, especially if they are to take place consistently. Walking through this important aspect, and even role-playing salon greetings, are important exercises when establishing a higher ritual of care.

Making people feel welcome, and the pleasure provided by beautiful details as they enter your business, are incredibly powerful elements in romancing and retaining your clientele. Fresh air is a must even though it can be a challenge in a busy salon environment. Providing current magazines, a sparkling appearance, a comfortable temperature, and tasty refreshments are all part of the details that provide a sincere "hello." When stylists augment this great beginning by escorting their clients to their next stop in the service process, an extraordinary greeting is complete. More great enticements for clients to remain with your business!

Working toward a better welcome for clients is an ongoing process that begins with the awareness of it's importance and the role every salon member can play in making clients feel well cared for. Each person, in their own way, is responsible for creating a great visit for every client who enters your business. By committing to great care and following through with action, your salon will have mastered a potent step in your contemporary client care program.

3. Running on Time

Discussing this important part of your contemporary client care program can be done at any time. However, it might be wise to refrain from seriously working on changing behavior in this area until the cleanliness factor in your salon has significantly improved. Pushing your staff to make too many changes at once can often create a hostile backlash.

Initial conversations about being punctual can emphasize the importance of a timely service as well as the detrimental behavior that comes from being chronically late. Once you are ready to focus on this matter, group and individual talks can become much more specific. The first thing you will want to make sure of is that you personally are not habitually late when arriving at the salon or caring for clients.

If you feel that a few minutes either way is not important, check with your front desk. They are the ones who must calm and reassure clients who are agitated because their stylists are not there to greet them. And when stylists arrive late, they cannot be prepared mentally or physically to draw on 100% of their abilities. It is a losing habit, and a very difficult one to overcome. The destruction to an individual's clientele, as well as damage to the salon's well-being, is substantial.

Some suggestions for changing chronically late behavior are:

+ An initial talk regarding their behavior and what it is doing to their career.
+ Discovering what their commitment truly is to changing this destructive habit.
+ Offering a change in schedule, if this would be helpful.
+ Helping to supervise their books if chronic lateness is related to not completing services on time during the day.

> The first thing you will want to make sure of is that you personally are not habitually late when arriving at the salon or caring for clients.

- Refraining from giving them new clients as first appointments if their problem is a timely arrival to work.
- Listening for solutions. Their suggestions in this area may be the best.
- Being willing to terminate their employment if you feel their behavior is harming your business.

The Habitually Late Story

An owner in Orange County, California, once shared that she had three stylists who lived approximately ten minutes from each other. Two arrived for work on time every day but the third stylist was always ten minutes late.

Exasperated by her constant excuses, the owner asked the tardy stylist why two other people who lived within ten minutes of her home never had any difficulties getting to work. Why couldn't she show up on time as well? The employee, with a very serious face, candidly responded, "But they live ten minutes closer. That's why they get here first. If I lived closer, I would be on time, too."

People who arrive habitually late for work do not have the sincere goal of arriving to work on time. It is a tough issue and one that you will need to weigh carefully. How important is being on time?

4. Pleasurable Acts

Pleasurable experiences can be the numerous details that you provide clients during their services or they can be more formal "extras" that everyone in your salon does each time clients visit. (See Chapter 9, "Acts of Pleasure" for more information about the nice details you can provide your clientele.) The ideas are endless and quite enjoyable to discuss with your entire group. Allowing staff creativity in offering suggestions will reveal new ideas every time pleasurable acts are discussed.

You will have your plate full for quite some time until everyone gets a firmer grip on the challenges of creating extraordinary client care. Yet, while working on mastering these necessary changes, you can begin adding many pleasurable moments for your clients without involving a lot of time or your staff. By strategically placing objects (a mirror, hand lotion, and hair spray in the restroom, for instance) or by improving your supplies (soft towels, attractive robes, and more), you will have the advantage of introducing pleasure into your salon visits from the beginning of your program. When the time is right and everyone has adapted to the previous steps of your circle of care, you can begin introducing this concept.

Regularly treating clients to extras that heighten their sense of beauty and well-being are gifts that never go unrewarded. Rituals of care make clients loyal and eager to return for their next appointment which is, in effect, also caring for

When your staff is ready and willing to accept the added responsibility of pleasurable care, bring in as many professionals as you possibly can to educate and structure their activities.

ourselves. Putting as many non-labor improvements in as soon as possible is a smart move. When your staff is ready and willing to accept the added responsibility of pleasurable care, bring in as many professionals as you possibly can to educate and structure their activities.

- ✦ Aromatherapy classes can educate your staff on the benefits and applications of these potent gifts of nature.
- ✦ Massage therapists are invaluable in establishing a prescribed method of massage during shampoos.
- ✦ Massage therapists can turn an ordinary pedicure or manicure into an extraordinary experience. Provide education for your nail technicians in this area and watch your nail business grow. (Be sure to promise your clients a massage that lasts a prescribed amount of time.)
- ✦ Re-read your beauty school textbook and re-learn how to do a great scientific brushing. It is healthy as well as pleasurable.
- ✦ Practice safe draping. Your staff can easily establish a prescribed draping method. Make sure you support their efforts by providing adequate, well-designed capes.
- ✦ Create other ways to make clients feel, as well as look, better because of their time spent with your salon.

5. Communication

Communication is an intricate skill not easily mastered without a considerable amount of education and discussion. These skills should be supported continuously with ongoing information. Outside educators skilled in this area are valuable to the success of everyone who belongs to your business and communication exercises and group studies are also helpful.

Communication is an intricate skill not easily mastered without a considerable amount of education and discussion.

LuLu Benavidez of LuLu The Salon in Galveston, Texas, has a seminar that offers classes to her people on a variety of subjects. It is structured as three partial days of learning per week for a period of one month each year. The seminars concentrate on personal development, communication, and trends. Not only does her staff learn the nuances of communication from teachers found at local universities, they also learn about body language and personality profiles. One year, Benavidez even featured an actor who was performing in a popular play. He taught her staff how to bring out different parts of their own personalities to match those of their clients.

Opportunities in the area of communication are endless and they are also fascinating to everyone attending the classes. While the information learned is mostly for clients, it also filters into the group dynamics of your salon. When staff members have fewer misunderstandings, they are much better bonded than those caught between rifts in the salon.

Michael Christopher Salon in Wilmington, Delaware, has a one-day retreat each year to reinforce group dynamics. "We learn better ways to talk to each other," states Michael Hemphill, owner, "and we constantly reinforce these things in our meetings. It's interesting to hear how differently our people relate to each other after one of these sessions. But, if you don't continue to review these teachings, the information will be lost within a few months. We reinforce our staff with motivational tapes and continuous discussions in our meetings."

Just as we should be striving toward better communication with our spouses and children, we also need to be working toward better communication with our clients and peers.

Relationships are complicated issues. Just as we should be striving toward better communication with our spouses and children, we also need to be working toward better communication with our clients and peers. Reading current books on relationships, and sharing highlights with your staff, also improve their skills. They are usually written in an entertaining style and are able to establish common ground with most people. There are numerous business books on client communication that can provide a lot of knowledge as well as pleasure from studying. Salon professionals are people oriented and love the intense interaction experienced when caring for the appearance of their clientele. Because of this, you will most likely find some of the best communication pupils in the world in your very own salon.

There are also companies that can provide speakers for your salon on a variety of subjects, including communication. There may be a local company specializing in this service within your own area. Check with your clients to see if anyone is a speaker or has an excellent referral for one. Also, ask Chambers of Commerce and local universities for referrals.

Once your staff has a better idea of good communication, you can begin creating points, or even an outline, of what your salon considers to be a quality consultation and when it should be used. Like other aspects of your program, creating a committee of salon members to research and make suggestions in this area is a good idea.

A consultation is a vital discovery process that allows accurate information to be exchanged between stylist and client. Rating high as an important factor in client satisfaction, skillfully interviewing clients and offering quality input about their appearance are extremely critical to a lasting business relationship. A thorough consultation should be done before any service is performed. Not only will it shed new light on a client's current state of mind, it will also give the stylist a good feeling on how their last service has been received. Beyond that, it can also help develop a client's total beauty image, increasing the number of services a client utilizes in your salon and building a rapport that encourages referrals. In most cases, a quality consultation supports the belief that most good clients are not found; they are created by those who take the time to enrich their lives by listening and giving knowledgeable suggestions.

Consultations offer a moment where stylists and clients can stop, talk, and develop a service strategy. It is also a process where key points are covered while the service is being performed.

Suggested elements of a consultation include:

+ Always asking open-ended questions.

+ Checking with clients to see if they were satisfied with their last service. How did they feel when they left? Did they successfully manage their style? Did it have the longevity they were looking for? Were they happy?

+ Are they looking for change? Do they have something in mind? Give professional suggestions on new styles that look great and are within their personal guidelines of care.

+ Sharing what services they would need to successfully achieve the look they want.

+ Informing them of added services and products that can enhance their total beauty: shine treatments, better haircare products, and even more timely appointments.

+ Providing ongoing communication during the service including styling tips (how-to's as well as versatility of the cut) and ways to better care for their hair, nails, or skin.

+ As always, once your consultation method has been created, put it in writing and regularly review this procedure with your staff. This serves to not only reinforce it's content, but also to change anything that is awkward or otherwise not working.

> All staff members should have a one-on-one meeting with management at least every three months.

The Ponytail Story

A man with very long hair went into a hair salon and asked for a haircut. The person taking care of him asked if he wanted to keep his ponytail. When he replied 'yes,' she expertly snipped it off and handed it to him. It was just a case of misunderstanding...

Often we use the same words but mean different things. Learning to communicate clearly, listening well, and taking the time to clarify information are all part of exceptional client care. Without these skills, we do not have the power to consistently please those who come to us for services.

6. Excellent Services

No matter how well you care for the details of client care, your salon must be performing at an above-average level in service quality or steady growth will remain elusive. Clients are intelligent creatures and they will know if they are getting the best at your salon, or if they should check out the hair company down the street.

Leading salons, like Gary Manuel, have established benchmarks of growth to teach and assess their staff's performance. Keeping track of your staff, and making sure they are maintaining current skills, cannot be stressed enough. All staff members should have a one-on-one meeting with management at least every three months. Not only can their performance be evaluated, but yours can as well. By doing so, services or attitudes that are slipping can be made productive once more before any real harm has been done. It also keeps you and your staff on a steady path toward success.

The first step to make sure this happens is a high-caliber educational program. Education is always an exciting experience. When selected wisely, it can also dramatically enhance the quality of all services performed in your salon. Always try to get as much hands-on training as possible. While you are doing it, carefully evaluate the person scheduled to conduct the class and get a step-by-step explanation of what will be covered. The programs should be challenging to your people. Hands-on participation is best, especially when taught by a teacher of both skill and experience.

Equally important is to put your educational program in writing and to make sure it also contains a balance of career development classes and business. How many classes are you going to host per year? How many total will be part of your program? Quality salons plan six months to a year in advance for their education. You should do the same. If, for some reason, your business takes another course, you can always add classes to reflect your new energies.

If your salon suffers from poor class attendance, it is important to discover why. Often, it is not lack of interest in furthering skills and knowledge, but rather the classes are simply not challenging enough to warrant much enthusiasm. Whatever the case, your salon must grow together in order to present a clear message to your clientele. Allowing staff to help with the agenda and having everyone agree to certain classes are very helpful when designing a program. If your staff is large and their experience varies, consider having basic classes optional. As Michael Hemphill says, "Some people don't need to learn how to comb hair anymore."

Good education can be costly. Classes that go beyond product knowledge and lectures by salon educators are usually not provided free by manufacturers, although you can earn some classes as a direct result of selling and promoting their products. The simple question "How much product do I have to purchase in order to have one of your platform members come to my salon and give a class at no charge?" will usually get the ball rolling. Once you find out, get your staff involved because they have the most power to sell products and recommend services.

Beyond freebies, however, there are many classes which you can purchase. The greatest challenge is not finding educational opportunities but funding them. As previously mentioned, the Gary Manuel Salon deducts $11.00 per paycheck to pay for advanced education courses. Many salons, such as Diva Studio, allow their stylists to purchase their education separately by established individually earned funds. But the most exciting educational program by far comes from a small salon in Massachusetts. Zona Salons of Norwell, MA, ties educational dollars into retail sales (matching percentages) as well as add-on services and new business. Frank Zona designed his program to reflect a percentage of sales from bowl treatments, lash and brow enhancements, as well as special services that are promoted at any given time, to go toward a stylist's education. He also credits staff when they bring in new business on their own. Their proceeds are used each year to fly to Europe for one week and attend an advanced academy. Their earnings pay for airfare, tuition fees, hotels, and food. Top that!

7. Prebooking

One of the most important yet most overlooked actions in the salon is prebooking. In fact, the majority of clients in our industry are leaving our salons without making their next appointment. Consider the following:

One of the most important yet most overlooked actions in the salon is prebooking.

- ✦ Discussing ways to overcome objections is very beneficial.
- ✦ Sharing salon reports is a sobering experience. Calculating lost revenues is also a jolt of reality that tends to motivate those who want to earn more money.
- ✦ Physically looking at the appointment books together to tally the current prebookings can also enhance your staff's desire to commit to books that reflect a healthy percentage of prebookings.
- ✦ Working with your front desk personnel to support stylists in their desire for higher prebookings is strongly suggested. Avoid any misunderstandings as to your intentions by sharing these methods with your staff.

Sincerely assure everyone who is taking this extra step that, as time goes by, prebooking becomes much easier to accomplish. Clients want convenience in their lives and part of that is being able to get their hair done when they want to. Because prebooking fills up books in advance, "what they want to" may not always be possible unless they reserve their time before leaving.

8. Follow-Through

Follow-through encompasses a range of acts that keep clients happy and anxious to return to your salon. Some of them can be instituted as soon as you have received the cooperation of your staff while others should be saved for a later date when the rest of your system is running successfully. Consider this range of follow-through techniques:

- One of the most basic forms of follow-through is a call to remind clients of their appointment. This practice saves thousands of dollars per year from no-shows. It is also a positive act which clients find thoughtful as well as professional.

- Simple follow-throughs also can be reminder calls to clients who are due in but do not have an appointment on the books. It is a positive act that also serves as an intermediate step to full prebooking. The difference is that a simple reminder call lets clients know their hair needs attention while only a prebooked appointment can give them the exact time and day they want to come in.

- Telephone calls by stylists, or the front desk three days after all chemical services are also professional acts that keep communication going between client and salon. The key to this act of follow-through is consistency.

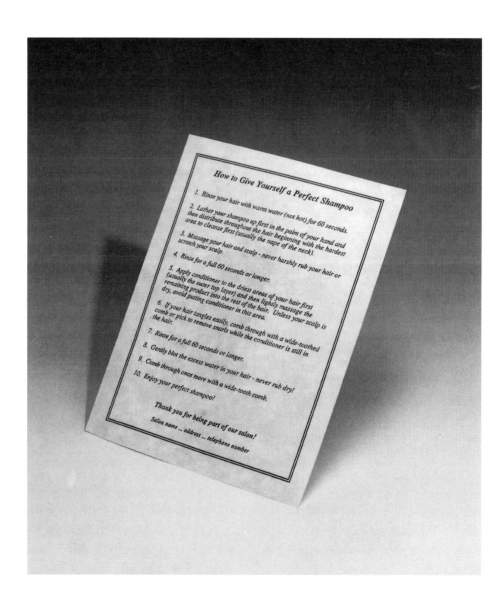

Figure 6-2
A "Perfect Shampoo"
flyer.

◆ Giving clients written instructions on how to care for their hair is also a great follow-through. When given at the end of the service, clients can leave feeling much more confident on how to care for their hair at home. Simple instructions, such as how to give their hair a perfect shampoo and conditioner are great. Seasonal instructions are also greatly appreciated and detailed steps on how to care for hair after chemical services is vital. Once this practice is instituted, you will find clients sharing things with you such as how they taped these instructions on the inside of the medicine chest so they would always have them or how they put them in plastic to keep them safe. It is a simple act of follow-through from the salon's perspective but a valuable service when viewed through the eyes of a client.

◆ Follow-through also means giving your clients recognition of their loyalty and worth to your salon. These follow-throughs can be in the form of verbal praise, thank-you notes, or gifts.

Training your staff to voice their appreciation is a big step in customer satisfaction. By perfecting your paperwork, your salon is in a good position to thank those who have referred other clients to your business. Gifts are also valuable tools of care. They can be complimentary salon visits, free add-on services, or even tangible gifts strategically given to boost the enthusiasm of your clientele

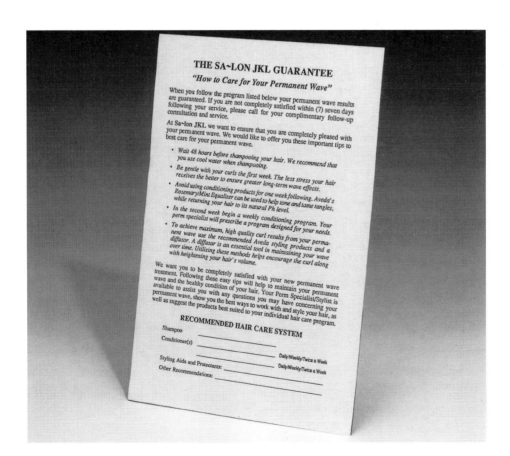

Figure 6-3
A permanent wave flyer. (Courtesy of Salon JKL.)

STAFF SURVEYS

While your salon program is evolving, it is essential to keep a pulse on the mind-set of your staff. One of the best ways to do this is to survey them. Staff surveys enable all members to voice their opinions, especially if they are reluctant to do so in front of others. Since good surveys offer the option of remaining anonymous, they can also be the most truthful. By creating surveys that allow your people to complain and offer their own solutions, you will have a much better chance of maintaining a cohesive group that holds similar ideals and goals.

Successful salons regularly poll their staff on a variety of issues. "How am I doing as a manager?" "What do your think of the salon?" "What suggestions do you have for improvement?" These are just some of the questions you can ask your people on a regular basis. But, to create a baseline for their opinions and feelings, it is very important to begin surveying your staff at the onset of your improvements.

Before making up your own staff survey, seriously think about what are the most important things you want to know during this phase of your program. Then ask about those issues. Do not be afraid of what you will hear. If some of the feedback is negative, try to turn these complaints into solutions for a better and stronger salon.

"We poll our staff every six months," Steven Brooks, owner of Diva Studio reveals. "I want to keep in touch with my people. Not only do I discover what they want from my salon, but also how I'm doing and ways we can all work together to make the whole thing an even bigger success."

While your salon program is evolving, it is essential to keep a pulse on the mindset of your staff. One of the best ways to do this is to survey them.

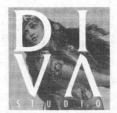

Staff Survey

1. What do you feel makes DIVA so special?

2. What are your 3 favorite qualities about DIVA?

3. What are your 3 least favorite aspects of DIVA?

4. How would you improve our customer service?

5. How would you improve our education program?

6. How would improve our TEAM morale?

7. What would you like to see more of at DIVA?

8. What would you like to see less of at DIVA?

9. What should we discontinue at DIVA?

10. If there is one thing you could change at DIVA what would it be?

11. What will you personally be focusing on to build your business at DIVA?

3159 W TOMPKINS, LAS VEGAS, NV 89103 - (702) 736-2011

Figure 6-4
A staff survey. (Courtesy of Diva Studio)

chapter 7

Creating a Contemporary Front Desk

HOTopic

1. Controlling the front desk environment
2. Image
3. Smooth check-ins and check-outs
4. Coding the appointment books
5. Supporting the circle of care

REDEFINING THE FRONT DESK

The role salon coordinators play in your business has expanded. Once called receptionists, their job has grown from simply answering phones and preparing coffee to co-managing specific areas of the salon. This chapter outlines many of the possibilities you have in defining the multiple roles of your front desk personnel. Whether you choose to implement all or just part of these suggestions, you will more fully develop your front-desk talent, greatly enhancing the image and performance of your salon.

By the time you have introduced your circle of care to your staff, your front desk will have already worked with you on many things which make up your entire contemporary client care program. They have been instrumental in creating complete salon records, and have become far more conscientious about your business environment. Because of these things, your salon coordinators have already made many improvements, proving themselves capable of participating in the changes that are yet to come.

ORGANIZATION OF TRAINING

There are four things you must do to create a contemporary front desk:

1. Establish a regular meeting schedule/format for your front desk. Receive their commitment of attendance.
2. Define the front desk image.
3. Work together to devise ways to work smart.

4. Establish the role of the front desk in your overall client care program including each step of your circle of care.

1. Establishing Meetings

Meetings with your front desk team should be done on a regular basis without the presence of your artistic staff. These private times give everyone the opportunity to speak more openly about the challenges they are facing as well as offer solutions that will enhance their ability to have maximum performance. Regarding the contemporary client care program, they can also concentrate more efficiently on their multiple responsibilities toward management, staff, and clients.

Meeting with your front desk team, and working through their involvement in your program, should be planned as carefully as your general staff meetings. Growing together, and giving plenty of time to evolve into a top-notch team will be a rewarding experience. Your front desk has a different mindset than your artistic team and it is likely that you will discover their concerns for success are very similar to your own.

2. Defining Image

One of your front desk's primary responsibilities is to visually, as well as verbally, communicate the spirit of your salon. If you are promoting cutting-edge fashion, your front desk staff needs to embody the beauty of your work in their own appearance. Stylists also must realize that it is their responsibility to make sure that salon coordinators wear their best creations. It is definitely a team effort. Front desk and general staff meetings are great times to reinforce your salon's policy on reflecting personal appearance.

Offering services for a very minimal charge to all salon coordinators will greatly enhance their ability to reflect the image you are expecting at the front desk. Including your salon coordinators in all classes and offering regular seasonal updates for their hair, makeup, skin and nails, are smart moves. They not only create a better front desk image, but also add to the numerous benefits you offer as part of their employment package. Giving your front desk staff personnel written service benefits, including when they may receive them, will also be a tremendous help. Establishing a written grooming standard gives all your staff an accurate idea of how they are to meet the expectations of the salon. Making this clear at the very beginning of employment can also eliminate a lot of misfires when hiring front desk personnel. People generally look their very best while interviewing for a job. If you do not make it clear that a groomed appearance is expected at all times, you might leave yourself open to some unpleasant surprises.

> Meetings with your front desk team should be done on a regular basis without the presence of your artistic staff.

The Dress-Up Story

A salon coordinator was hired partially because of her terrifically trendy appearance. Her hair was a great shade of burgundy, her make-up definitely on the cutting edge, and the clothes she wore reeked of Melrose, CA. The first day of work, however, she showed up with a puffy, plain face and a strained expression typical of someone who has overslept. She also wore a pair of pale blue vinyl house slippers she had forgotten to change before leaving home. The owner was not at the front desk to greet her immediately, and it was not until an hour and numerous clients later that she realized the newest member of her front desk team was caring for clients with her bright burgundy hair secured on top of her head with a chewed-up pencil. When confronted, the receptionist looked shocked and offended. No one had told her she was expected to dress up!

The moral of this story: Never assume. Beauty and fashion represent your livelihood. Protect them at all times!

3. Working Smart

There is also a great emphasis on working, as well as looking, smart. Doing business with your front desk can bring harmony or serve as a lesson in aversion therapy for your clients. By allowing your staff to create many of their structures, you will enable them to assume new attitudes with their positions. What do they think? How can they create better service? Salon coordinators understand all the problems associated with their jobs and will likely have the majority of the solutions. Just ask and listen!

Clients expect superb service and part of this is having a smooth check-in and a speedy check-out. By working with your front desk, these procedures can be revised and streamlined to meet, and even exceed, the expectations of your clientele.

Clients need to be checked-in in less than thirty seconds after being greeted. Even when clients are purchasing retail products, the check-out procedure should take an absolute maximum time of three minutes. If your salon is not meeting these superb service requirements, work on your procedures until they are effortlessly accomplished.

One of the best ways to ensure that this happens is to be completely prepared to conduct business each day. This means having enough change to take care of all sales and dealing with credit cards only through on-line services that can process and approve charges within seconds of requests. Keeping check information on file for regular clients also speeds up the check-out process.

> Even when clients are purchasing retail products, the check-out procedure should take an absolute maximum of three minutes.

Even preparing beverages can slow down client handling time. At the start of each day, small time-savers like pre-filling coffee filters and having extra cups set out along with the condiments so that clients can help themselves to salon refreshments helps a lot during busy times.

Having your products properly coded prior to stocking is an enormous time saver. By utilizing a bar code/scanning system, you can speed up the process even more. Also, establish a policy of who is responsible for gathering retail products for clients prior to check-out. Is it the front desk or stylists?

Electronic appointment books have faster capabilities for managing salon bookings. They can provide computerized waiting lists to efficiently re-fill canceled appointments and also generate service tickets, eliminating hundreds of hours each year spent creating and processing these slips by hand. They are also much faster when changing appointments, and a week of their bookings can be put on the screen at one time to facilitate a faster booking time for clients making their next appointment.

4. Embracing the Circle of Care

Your front desk also plays important roles in your circle of care. They often act as the core of your plan, keeping the circle of care intact and running smoothly. Your first step in including them in this portion of your program is to give your salon coordinators the power to control their environment. Once they have full authority to manage these areas, positive first impressions of your business will grow a quantum leap.

Cleanliness
Their milieu normally includes the waiting room, retail area, and front desk. A big part of that impression is the cleanliness (including orderliness) of all the areas they control. Clients sit in the waiting area drinking beverages and physically touching the front desk. Make sure that what they are coming in contact with is reassuring and clean.

Your front desk personnel must first be made aware of the exact nature of their responsibility. If retail shelves are to be kept in top-notch order, they need to know exactly what this means. Once they realize what is expected, they can set up a cleaning schedule that fits sensibly into their busy days.

Stocking is the same. When are the shelves replenished? What are the policies on products? Are they restacked during the day as supplies are depleted? Who is responsible for keeping the stock in order and how important is this? If well-organized retail shelves rate high in your salon, the importance of maintaining them must be communicated to your front desk staff.

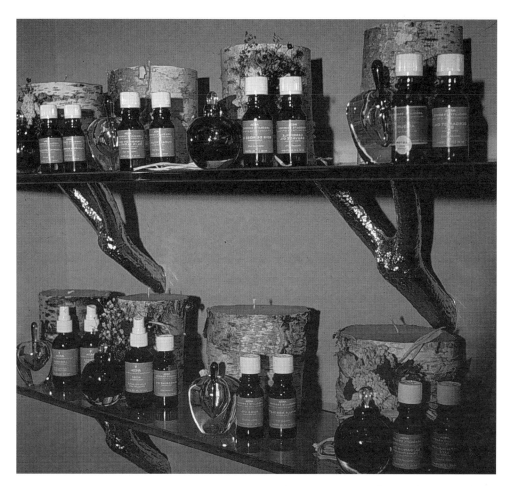

Figure 7-1
A retail display area.
(Courtesy of Aruj Salon
& Spa)

There is also the issue of the refreshment area. What types of refreshments should be available? Balancing the tastes of your clientele with issues of cleanliness is important in maintaining an attractive center. Your front desk can organize light snacks and drinks and they should set up their own procedures on how to care for them. Also included is the importance of not having your entire staff use this area for their own consumption. Cleaning up after clients is one thing, but constantly cleaning up after staff members will understandably create anger and resentment among your front desk personnel. Having a refreshment center in the staff's break area is a better alternative. There, they can consume, enjoy, and clean up after themselves.

The front desk should be wiped down regularly either as part of closing or opening your salon. Ink smears, hand prints, and general grime appear quickly and can make even a beautiful salon appear shabby and unkempt. Your front desk personnel need to set up a schedule to care for the front desk as well as a policy regarding any front areas that need attention throughout the day. Make sure you supply them with the proper cleaning supplies to do the job quickly and efficiently.

Clutter is also a big issue. Magazines must have a place along with a commitment to keep them there, no matter how many times the waiting area needs to be straightened each day. Magazine receptacles work wonders in this seemingly uphill battle for a neat, orderly waiting area. Also, keeping loose literature to a minimum will prevent your reception area from quickly looking like a parking lot on a windy day.

Everything within the front desk environment should also be organized and maintained by your salon coordinators, ranging from how your beverage center is set up to the maximum age of your magazines. With their dedication and your guidance, your salon can present a beautiful image to your clientele every day you are open for business.

The first step to a beautiful front area is to get physically organized. Work with your salon coordinators to establish a place for everything right down to the scratch pads. If tossing pencils and pens around the desk is a habit, or magazines are askew for hours, work with them until these habits disappear. If staff members are still invading their space, have them stop as well.

Your front desk personnel should also itemize everything they need to run a tight ship, and you need to make sure they have it in good supply. Chasing forms, searching for products, and scouring the salon for paper clips takes time away from what is important—caring for your business.

Welcome
Every client who walks through your door should receive a warm greeting within thirty seconds of their arrival. If your front desk staff is busy on the telephone or with other clients, teach them the art of eye contact and non-verbal acknowledgment. If you think this is too stringent, think about the number of times you have been out shopping and put merchandise back on the shelf because there was no salesperson there to help you. Or, think of the businesses you have entered and immediately left because you were not recognized when you came in. Your clients, no matter how many times they have visited your salon, need to know they are welcome and will be immediately cared for by your staff. If they have to approach the front desk to ask if their stylist knows they are there, or even sit quietly without acknowledgment, your front desk is not doing their job.

Affording your salon coordinators the opportunity to work through their own scenarios of poor service will serve as boosters for their own sensitivity to clients. It is a great way to teach them that during their time at work, it is not about what they are doing but how the client is feeling that is important. In this regard, role playing can be invaluable. Even exercises of time serve as lessons in the importance of immediate service.

Every client who walks through your door should receive a warm greeting within thirty seconds of their arrival.

Exercises in Time

Allow your staff to share their feelings after each step of this exercise. Did they feel important, unimportant, or neglected?

- ✦ Stand at the front desk, purse or briefcase in hand, for thirty seconds with personnel moving about, not recognizing your presence.
- ✦ Stand at the front desk, purse or briefcase in hand, for one minute under the same conditions.
- ✦ Stand at the front desk, purse or briefcase in hand, for three minutes under the same conditions.

Dispositions sour quickly as seconds tick by. Eye contact coupled with a simple nod works wonders during busy times.

There is always the importance of smiling. Surprisingly, this expression often takes practice, especially when things become stressful. It is easy to smile when the phones are quiet and the salon is not full of clients but what about times during the day when telephones go ballistic, people are piled up at the front desk, and others are coming through the door eager to say "hello" to a happy receptionist? Will their expectations be met? Make sure your front desk personnel is aware of the importance you place on this friendly expression and practice it yourself.

Also, frustration of any kind does not belong in the workplace. If you find one of your front desk personnel becoming stressed, do not hesitate to intervene. Make sure they understand that asking for front desk assistance in order to take a break and re-balance is perfectly okay. Staff problems are not welcomed by clients no matter how sympathetic they may seem. And nothing justifies unkind words, angry gestures, or disgruntled attitudes on the part of your staff.

Also, concentrate on things that help your salon coordinators radiate their message. Be up front to greet clients yourself whenever possible. Fresh flower displays are beautiful in this respect and can often be bartered with a local florist. A basket of freshly-dried potpourri at the desk is a wonderful hello. Also, creative displays and cheerful signage can heighten your overwhelming message of "Welcome to our salon!"

Running on Time

The front desk has a two-edged responsibility on issues of "running on time." First, they need to be efficient with their own handling procedures so clients are ready to be greeted by their stylists on a timely basis. They also have to know which stylists are running on time and which are not. Regarding the latter, if it is just a few minutes, a few words to clients when they enter help soothe frustrations. If a stylist is running fifteen minutes late or longer, informed salon

If you find one of your front desk personnel becoming stressed, do not hesitate to intervene.

coordinators can make courtesy calls to let clients know there will be a delay in receiving their service.

There are also important issues of opening and closing the salon. The big priority in your business is to be fully prepared each day when you open your doors. Working through systems that ensure that the salon will be left in an acceptable condition in the evening, as well as ready for business the next morning, make this important criteria possible.

If your salon does not have a maid or shop assistant, all areas that are directly managed by the front desk also need to be maintained by them. Go over your "morning greeter" list with your front desk personnel and allow them to devise a schedule that ensures that their area is sparkling fresh by the time of opening each day.

Also, there is the issue of booking times. Yielding to client pressures to "squeeze them in" contributes to chaos in a stylist's schedule. Your salon coordinators are in control of this situation, and can help redirect clients to other days and times as well offer them waiting list status. Standing firm on this issue will save thousands of lost dollars each year due to over-compressed scheduling.

Pleasurable Acts
Pleasurable acts by the front desk can come in the form of gifts and samples, thank you notes, refreshments, the strategic diffusion of essential oils, or soothing music. It can also be something as simple as always keeping a jar of colorful candy or a basket of fresh apples at the front desk. As your ability to provide more pleasurable acts for your clients increases, your front desk's participation will as well. Let them know they will be part of this endeavor and keep them informed of your plans as they evolve. Planning, scheduling, and mutual participation are all factors of success when creating acts of pleasure for your clientele.

Communication
Communication is a complicated issue for salon coordinators who must be skilled on many different levels. Clients need information as well as service. Plus, a large percentage of all types of business information is funneled through the front desk.

Salon coordinators must be able to communicate clearly to clients regarding their appointments, available salon services and products, as well as future commitments. They need to know how to voice concern when it is warranted and praise whenever possible. Every word they utter must be done in an extremely pleasant manner.

> **Yielding to client pressures to "squeeze them in" contributes to chaos in a stylist's schedule.**

To make their jobs even more important, front desk personnel must also be able to talk to a wide variety of artistic personalities, helping them at all times throughout their busy days. Plus, they need to get along amongst themselves. All of this must be accomplished while maneuvering in tight quarters—not easy!

There is also one other very important issue. Your front desk personnel must be able to talk to clients about services and products, including selling them. To keep your salon healthy and salaries high, front desk personnel should be able to generate enough sales each week to pay at least 50% of their salaries. Is this a revolutionary thought? Actually, it is a practical concept.

One of the most desirable types of people you can hire is someone who has worked behind the cosmetic counters in department stores. They have been taught how to sell-through to the client and they know the importance of a pleasant, helpful personality. They are accustomed to creating accurate, detailed paperwork and most have had exposure to computers. To them, selling is not a dirty word; it is simply part of good service.

Without this attitude, much of what you offer your clients will remain a mystery. Your artistic staff has a narrow focus and will share only a small amount of what you actually carry. Front desk personnel have a much broader scope of your salon. Support them with signage whenever possible, and offer specials they can present to clients. Above all, hire those who enjoy selling as well as caring for your people. It is a smart move.

Including your salon coordinators in all classes regarding communication is an excellent step in the right direction. Working with people individually who have experienced problems due to miscommunication is another good way to help people speak and be understood. Salesmanship classes are also essential. Many people can talk about products, but most need education on how to finalize the sale.

Excellent Services

Excellent service at the front desk sets the standard for your entire salon. Treating clients importantly, giving great hospitality, and showing concern create more than a positive mood in the waiting area. These acts of great care also spill over into the rest of your salon.

Embodying many aspects already covered, as well as all points of the circle of care, excellent service by the front desk creates a smooth, efficient hub in your business, promoting trust and generating dollars throughout all the diverse levels of your business.

> **To keep your salon healthy and salaries high, front desk personnel should be able to generate enough sales each week to pay at least 50% of their salaries.**

Prebooking

Commitment to prebooking rests primarily on the shoulders of your stylists. They are in the position to make prebooking personally important to their clientele. However, your front desk people can act as essential team members by supporting your stylists' suggestions.

One of the easiest ways for salon coordinators to prebook clients is for stylists to designate on their service ticket the suggested number of weeks until their client's next visit. Stylists still need to tell clients verbally when they should come back and why. With a quick glance at their service ticket, salon coordinators can then support their advice by encouraging the client to commit to a date and time. For example, "Mrs. Jones, Alex has indicated that you should have your hair done again in five weeks. Let's take a peek at the books and see what is available."

Overcoming prebooking objections is also important training for your front desk personnel. Role playing among themselves in this respect works wonders. They have probably already heard every objection in the book, and by working together, they can diffuse them and commit your clients to their next visits. As more clients begin prebooking, it will become harder for those who are not prebooking to get the time and date preferred. Eventually, 80% or more of your salon clientele will prebook regularly. Like everything else, it simply takes time.

To help your stylists easily view how they are doing with their prebookings, code your books when someone prebooks by writing "PB" next to their name. Because stylists are visual people, placing a specific colored dot (small circular sticker) next to their name will vividly show everyone's prebookings.

Follow-Through

Follow-through by the front desk can range from creating a call list and confirming appointments, to making happiness calls after chemical services. It can also entail sending birthday cards, anniversary notes, and even flowers to deserving clientele. For those clients who simply will not make a prebooking, have your front desk personnel maintain a formal call list. If you do not have a computerized program for reminders, use a small binder and divide the book into weekly sections using standard notebook tabs. Using the designated return time on the service ticket, put these clients' names and telephone numbers on the week they are due in for services. Then, set up an official day each week to contact them. It works wonders!

In addition to creating call lists for clients, the front desk also has the responsibility of confirming all appointments. This professional service is appreciated by clients and eliminates the majority of no-shows on your books. For clients who

---

To help your stylists easily view how they are doing with their prebookings, code your books when someone prebooks by writing "PB" next to their name.

are online, e-mail confirmations are also a great way to remind them of their upcoming appointments.

To ensure that there are no misunderstandings with this procedure, you should consider coding confirmations on your books. Once accustomed to reminder calls, clients rely heavily on them to remember their appointments and when they do not receive a reminder, friction can be created between stylists, clients, and the front desk. A simple coding system can be devised by you and your front desk personnel to let everyone know the status of all confirmed appointments. The following suggested codes can be put next to clients' names as confirmation calls are being made.

C—Confirmed (talked directly to the person)

LM—Left message

EM—E-mail

By coding the books, your salon coordinators can see more readily if a reminder call has been missed. To further enhance accuracy as well as ease of reading, these codes should be written in red ink.

Within three days after chemical services are received (especially all perms and new color services), and after first-time visits, clients should be contacted to make sure they are happy with their visit. This procedure is a wonderful tool for client retention and needs to be practiced consistently by your salon. Clients leave salons for the smallest reasons—at least from the point-of-view of salon professionals. A perm that is slightly dry on the ends, bangs that are 1/4-inch too short, or blonde that has a hint more gold than expected can make even loyal clients withdraw from your salon. A simple phone call will remedy 90% of these minor complaints, and keep your clientele from silently seeking other salons for service.

If stylists make these calls, the gesture is extremely caring in the eyes of clients. However, because they often have an emotional bond with these stylists, the truth may not always be revealed. If your front desk makes these phone calls, they may receive more honest answers and be able to offer real help in the form of re-booking to remedy any problems. Either way, the primary concern is consistency. Whoever is in charge of the happiness calls for your salon must make sure they are done faithfully. A regular follow-up by you will also be instrumental in keeping this client-saving procedure alive.

Once you institute a "missing client" program, your front desk personnel will be involved in working toward retrieving clients who have drifted from your business. Included in this specialized program is producing, editing, and mailing literature appropriate to your program. Managing mailing lists and editing them with your stylists takes time and care. If your front desk personnel can

In addition to creating call lists for clients, the front desk also has the responsibility of confirming all appointments.

handle this job in terms of time, they will be the best people to do the job because they know your entire clientele far better than anyone else in your salon—including yourself! (For more information on client retrievals, see Chapter 10, "The Art of Retrieval.")

chapter 8

Rewarding
Your Clientele

HOTopic
1. System of appreciation
2. Gathering gifts
3. Goodwill gifting programs
4. The welcome packet
5. New client incentives and rewards
6. Circle of friends program

SYSTEM OF APPRECIATION

A good contemporary client care program includes recognition and reward for everyone frequenting your business. Developing programs that include presents, free services, and earned privileges are just some of the ways salons can invest in themselves while giving to others.

+ Select items and services that have good value but cost little or no money.

+ Your staff must understand the intention behind each reward.

+ A presentation method needs to be developed so that clients understand that the gifts you are giving them have value and that you are giving them as a symbol of appreciation by your salon.

+ Because your business is unique, you will also need to customize this program to suit your special needs.

We all feel our spirits lift when someone presents us with a gift. Whether it is an elaborate present or a simple flower, the very act inspires happiness and joy. Choosing the right words will create a present filled with value and goodwill. A note saying "Thank you for being part of our salon" means so much more than an item tossed into a bag without explanation or care.

Training staff members to treat salon gifts with as much value as you do, however, can be challenging. There are many things to cover when a client is with their stylist. Caught up in the rush, it is very tempting to hand something to somebody without a quality presentation. When appreciation is given in this fashion, there is little romance for the client and certainly no benefit to the

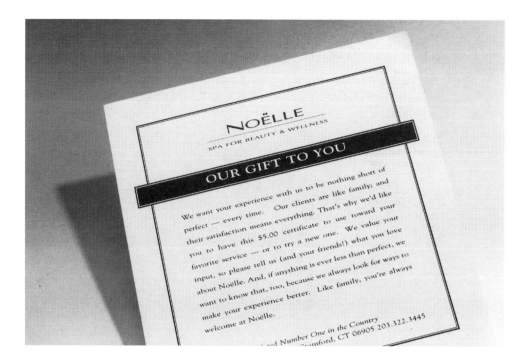

Figure 8-1
Client gift certificate.
(Courtesy of Noëlle
Spa for Beauty and
Wellness)

salon. Your program will be handled more consistently if the responsibility of presenting gifts is left to your front desk. It is very easy at the end of an appointment to check someone out, offer a prebooking, and give them a thank-you that includes more than a smile.

If the gift involves a service, however, it may still be important to have your stylists involved. Technical judgment and explanations are often needed in this area. By training your staff, and creating signage that will serve to both remind and announce your current program, you will have better opportunities to consistently service everyone's clients.

Gathering Your Gifts

Gifts come in many packages. You may choose to give away travel sizes of products you want to promote, or to offer a free service designed to enhance the salon experience. Buying and thinking ahead will enable you to give generously with little or no cost involved.

Manufacturers periodically have specials offering two products for the price of one. It could be two of the same product, or one free product when you buy another. If the products are of value to your business, buy as much as you possibly can afford. Part of your "free" goods can be sold for increased retail profits. Another portion may be kept packaged "as is" for purchasing incentives. But, at least one-third should be retained for "gifts only." Store these items where they will not disappear until you decide to use them as part of one of your gift promotions. When distributed with care, they will act not only as rewards for

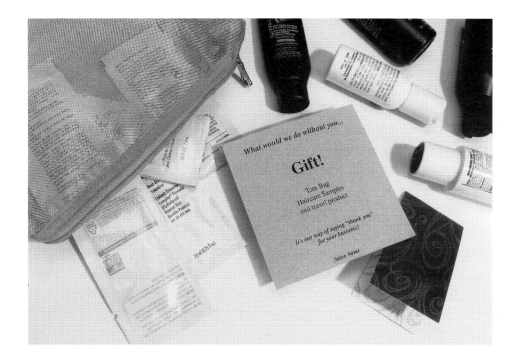

Figure 8-2
Client gift bag.

your clients, but also help to increase future retail sales. Often, leading manufacturers will offer a "free gift with purchase" special. These are great deals and not uncommon to find. Save these free gifts until you have enough products for a gift promotion (see ideas later in this chapter). The best way to find out about these specials, as well as many other deals, is to give sales reps the opportunity to sit down with you and explain their promotional opportunities. Make formal meetings with these people, limit their time to fit within your schedule, and listen. They have a lot to offer and much of it is below wholesale price!

The goal of partnering is for manufacturers and distributors to work more closely with salons. One of the best ways they can do this is to participate in your programs as well as their own. Once you have designed a gifting program for your clients, it would be very wise to have meetings with sales representatives (and, if you feel strongly about it, their managers) to share your programs with them. Becoming involved by supplying products for gifts is a great way to build their business as well as yours. You will find that some companies are willing to participate while others are not. Their attitudes should be carefully weighed before further deepening your commitment to their products. Just as your clients want romance, value, and benefits, you should expect the same. You are also a client and have all the same needs and wants as the people who walk through your door. Building is expensive, but being built is very profitable. The businesses you support should reflect this wisdom. Consider the following:

- Do your manufacturers have products that "sell themselves" or are product promotions necessary in order to be successful with their line?
- Gifts of popular products further enhance salon sales. Introducing a lesser known product from such a line is smart marketing.
- Gifts from lines that have little consumer recognition, however, should be carefully selected to include only the fastest moving items. Broad appeal is best.

Many manufacturers are now making guest artists available to their larger accounts for more than staff education. They are also available on a limited basis to educate and service your clientele. Examples of how you can use this talent bank freely are:

- If you carry a cosmetic line, there are professional companies that will provide you with a free "guest" makeup artist to work with your clientele for a specified amount of hours each season. Not only do they provide an exciting service but they also introduce new products, often come with gifts of their own, and sell your cosmetics without costing you a dime. These appearances can be billed as special events and even include special no-charge appointments for your clientele.
- Likewise, companies offering special backbar products, masks, hair treatments and more, will essentially do the same. All you have to do is ask!
- Organize an evening seminar for your clients on fashion, makeup, or hairstyles and many manufacturers will supply free guest speakers for these events! Client seminars are custom programs that are created upon demand—especially if you are a valued customer or have the potential of becoming one.

One note of warning, however: It is very important that all guest artists demonstrate the result and not the product. Although it is usually not perceived as such by company representatives, you never want your clients to feel like they are being subjected to the "big hustle." A product demonstration is not a free beauty seminar; it is a sales presentation. On the other hand, the knowledge gained from the demonstration of the product *is* valuable. Usually, when people like what they feel, see, or touch, they will want to take it home without prompting. So relax, be generous, and allow your clients to do the same. Simple joy in sharing the experience is all that is needed to create success.

Be very specific with any new company you are dealing with. Before ever purchasing a new line of products for your salon, have a meeting with the people in charge of making decisions. Take the time to share your programs with your potential new supplier and make very sure that they will be able to participate in your plans. Put your programs, and their promises, in writing. It will clarify your relationship, and keep it intact when your supplier has a change in personnel.

It is very important that all guest artists demonstrate the result and not the product.

Also, when negotiating gifts for your clients, do not forget to include samples. Many companies are cutting back on expenses by not supplying free samples in the quantities you may need for your programs. The best way to receive the amount you require is to share your philosophy of presentation and purpose. For example, "We always share our gifts with our clients and explain their purpose, benefits, and instructions for use. It is a planned presentation designed to create profit and success." Having a good purchase record with their company is also an important key in this matter, and by negotiating samples based on the amount you buy is a good way to ensure that they will continue to be supplied. Samples can be used traditionally to introduce a new product or to revive an old one. They can also be used as part of gift packs, which are explained later in this chapter.

Trade shows are wonderful places to find specials that fit nicely into most gifting programs, and many distributors have advance notice of the show deals they will be presenting. Try to get as much of this pre-show information as possible. Shows are usually very busy and can be confusing, to say the least. Many distributors will allow you to order just before or right after a trade show. Doing this outside the selling arena is often easier. But, the main point is to not miss the deals!

GOODWILL GIFTING PROGRAMS

At least two times a year, take the opportunity to thank all clients who frequent your shop by bestowing them with a gift. Recommended to last at least two weeks, these events can be promoted ahead of time to enhance business. If the gift is a product, pick one that you would like to introduce, or one that is already a winner. If it is a service, make sure it is appropriate for the season.

Product Gifts

All product gifts should be accompanied by a gift slip offering the client a discount on full-size products of the same brand. The offer should expire forty-five days after the slips are presented to the client. Each of the following suggestions can represent one complete gift, or you may opt to combine several of them for more impressive offerings.

- ✦ Travel products with case.
- ✦ One piece of makeup from your newest cosmetic collection.
- ✦ Hair brush with sample packets of hair care products.
- ✦ Facial brush with sample packets of skin care products.
- ✦ Loofah with facial care certificate.
- ✦ Bronzing powder with gift slip for cosmetics.

> At least three times a year, take the opportunity to thank all clients who frequent your shop by bestowing them with a gift.

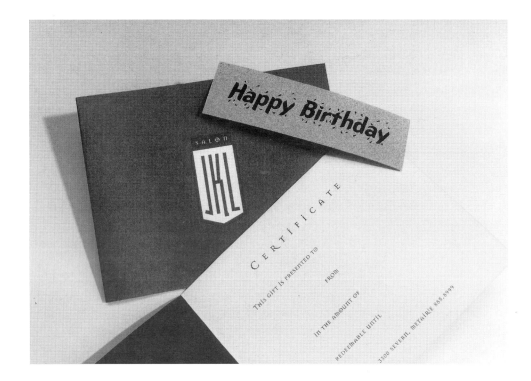

Figure 8-3
Client birthday gift
certificate. (Courtesy
Salon JKL)

✦ Small bottle of moisturizing shampoo with conditioner sample packets.

✦ Small bottle of custom-blended color enhancing shampoo.

✦ Complimentary makeup lesson with new collection.

✦ Re-mineralizing hair treatment.

✦ Translucent color service.

✦ Skin hydrating treatment.

Give beautifully as well as generously. Put your gifts together with attractive wrappings to enhance their value and delight the eye. As for manpower to accomplish this, do not forget to include your stylists. Making them a part of this program is as important as the program itself.

It is a great idea to send cards and reserve gifts for clients who are celebrating their birthdays. You can put together a gift bag that they may pick up during the week of their birthdays. Offering clients a free style during their birthday week is also a solid goodwill gesture. Not only are these gifts kind and thoughtful, they also encourage your clients to visit your salon one extra time during the year. Suggestions for a birthday bag include:

✦ Skin care samples.

✦ Hair care samples.

✦ Travel size product.

✦ A brush.

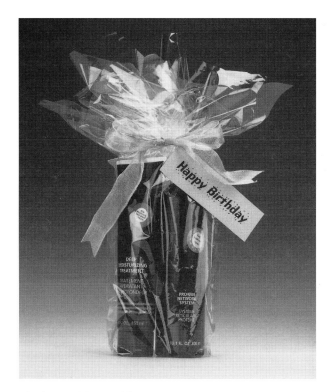

Figure 8-3a
Retail birthday gift.

Rewarding High-Dollar Clients

A positive way to end a substantial salon visit is with a gift. It could be a service gift designed to pamper and reward a client, or a product gift which would be particularly useful to them. Establish a criteria, explain it to your salon coordinators, and then follow up to make sure that those who deserve special tokens of appreciation receive them. For instance, for every $100.00 spent on services, a gift slip could be issued giving these clients a complimentary manicure, scalp treatment, or even a neck and shoulder massage during their next regularly scheduled visit.

Clients who choose to purchase products from your salon also deserve your appreciation. You can demonstrate your gratitude and give them incentives to continue buying from your company in the future. For a purchase of $50.00 or more (strictly in retail products) for instance, your salon coordinator could give them a gift slip for their next purchase: "Thank you, Mrs. Smith, for coming to see us. Here is a $5.00 gift slip toward your next purchase of products with our salon. Thanks again!"

Gifts from Salon Personnel

If you are building a nail or skin care business, the best opportunity to bond with a potential client is to create opportunities to experience one of these services. An excellent way to introduce new skin and nail care technicians is to offer a gift of their services to clients who are already booked for extensive

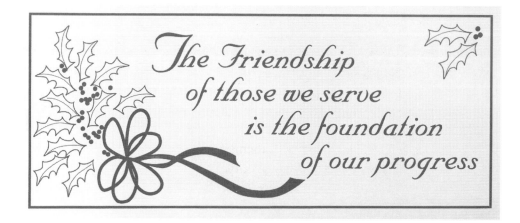

Figure 8-4
Christmas card.
(Courtesy Bob Steele
hairdressers)

chemical services. This will reward those spending the most in your salon and also give your technicians the opportunity to meet clients who are already utilizing multiple services. Offer a neck and shoulder massage, a paraffin treatment, or no-frills facial. Offer a skin softening treatment for the hands, a reflexology hand and forearm massage with essential oils, a complete manicure, or any other creation that you can conceive of that does not involve a great deal of time or expense. Whatever you decide, make sure it is actually offered as a legitimate service on your menu. Otherwise, it is clearly a marketing ploy and not a bonafide gift.

These types of gifting programs are extremely effective, but must be timed carefully to succeed. For instance, you would not want your manicurists to do a gifting program at the same time the salon was offering your bi-annual rewards program for your general clientele. You do not want your clients bombarded with an overload of goodwill; you want your front desk to be able to support and concentrate on one program at a time. Then, everyone's investment has a better opportunity to achieve profitable results.

NEW CLIENT INCENTIVES

Finding new clients is a very expensive proposition. Even though experts claim that it takes approximately $45.00 to attract a new client, this figure can be misleading. Anyone who has purchased advertisement knows that a $500.00 ad often yields only one or two new clients. Finding methods to create new clients without purchasing advertisements is vital to building your business. Then, after new clients have entrusted themselves in your care, you also need to devise numerous ways to retain their loyalty.

Referrals

Your existing clientele base is the richest source of new business you possess, and also the least expensive to cultivate. Many successful salons turn to their clients for growth, asking for new business and offering rewards in return. Carefully track the source of your new clients and send thank you notes and gifts to those who have thoughtfully recommended them to your business.

> **Your existing clientele base is the richest source of new business you possess**

Bob Steele, owner of Bob Steele Hairdressers in Atlanta, Georgia, calls these client recommendations "warm referrals." He has discovered that not only is it far more cost effective in attracting new people, but there is greater than a 50% chance of retaining them over "cold referrals" created by advertisements. They send gift certificates to all clients who refer new people to them throughout the year. They also have an annual referral campaign that offers rewards for sending "warm" referrals their way. Every December, this innovative salon sends beautifully embossed holiday cards out to their entire client database. Enclosed are two gift certificates—one for the client and another for a friend. During the months of January and February, when business normally slows down, the Bob Steele Hairdressers salon receives over three hundred new clients. This number increases as each new client responding to the campaign is also given incentives to refer new business. This one program produces approximately $70,000 annually in new business for the Bob Steele Hairdressers salon. It could work for your salon, too. "We believe in giving back to our clientele," shares Steele. "And, the best way to do that is to reward our loyal clients who actively promote our company. It is a profitable investment that generates revenues and happiness for everyone involved in our salon."

The Welcome Packet

Once clients have arrived at your salon, it is important to introduce them to all the services your salon has to offer, and to give them incentives to experience them. This can be awkward to accomplish in one sitting. In fact, in most cases, it takes several months to discover everything a salon has to offer. In the meantime, clients may be going elsewhere to receive those same services. Or,

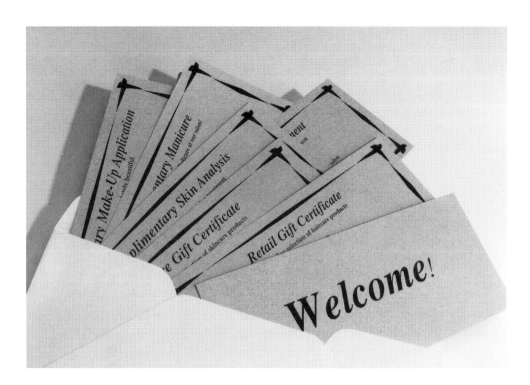

Figure 8-5
Welcome packet.

worse yet, they may leave because it is more convenient to get everything done elsewhere. Imagine that!

As a huge welcome to everyone who is new to your salon, and as a way to take your clients through the most important things you have to offer, you can organize your own "Welcome Packet" program. It is by far the greatest money maker your salon can invest in, and the best piece of goodwill you have at your disposal. A Welcome Packet contains gift slips for a variety of services. With these slips, you not only want people to try all your services, but to invest in them as well. The Welcome Packet is an entirely different approach from other gifts you offer your clients.

Gifts from the Welcome Packet are unearned and incomplete. That is, new clients who have not had the opportunity to be loyal to your salon are given dollars off towards a variety of services. The Welcome Packet is efficiently designed to create full-service clients in far less time than it would otherwise take. A Welcome Packet could contain gift slips reflecting:

✦ $10.00 towards the purchase of a facial.

✦ $5.00 towards the purchase of any skin care item.

✦ Free make up application with the purchase of any service.

✦ $5.00 towards the purchase of cosmetics.

✦ $5.00 towards the purchase of a manicure.

✦ $10.00 towards the purchase of a pedicure.

- ✦ $10.00 towards the purchase of a full weaving.
- ✦ $10.00 towards the purchase of a color-shine treatment.
- ✦ $10.00 towards the purchase of a permanent wave.
- ✦ An 8 oz. shampoo with their first haircut.

By offering the discounted nail services separately instead of lumping both into a $15.00 nail gift certificate, for instance, the manicurist is making a small amount of money on each service. Because there is money involved, people generally will not take advantage of these services unless they are interested in using them again in the future. So, despite the discount, there is a better chance that the client will be a repeat customer—especially if they are extremely pleased with their service.

For the stylist, it not only encourages chemical appointments, but also allows them to introduce additional services such as shine treatments that might otherwise remain unnoticed on the salon menu.

The Welcome Packet may be as simple as gift slips put in a plain envelope (which would cost less than 25 cents per set) or as elaborate as custom holders (such as those used for airline tickets), which would make the cost of the Welcome Packet range in price from $1.00 to $1.50 per set. Somewhere inbetween may be more practical. You can diminish the cost and increase your presentation by simply using nice envelopes, professionally printed with, "Welcome!" in large, open letters.

Custom packets are a necessity when creating a large selection of gifts. Most stylists, for instance, would not want a perm gift slip put in a packet for a new client who is already on the books for that service. On the other hand, if their current booking does not conflict with your content selection, never try and second guess what a client may or may not be interested in. Give them the packet in its entirety. In many instances, their choice of Welcome Packet services will surprise you!

> Welcome Packets should be presented by a trained person who can take the time to share, describe, and recommend each service contained in the packet.

Welcome Packets should be presented by a trained person who can take the time to share, describe, and recommend each service contained in the packet. The best candidate would be your salon coordinator. As a back up, you should have at least one other person who is trained and available to do this most important service. The salon owner can be the key player in this area. It is very impressive for a new client to be welcomed into the salon by an owner bearing gifts. It makes them feel important and the presentation will certainly be done to perfection!

For the receptionist, getting vital information for the client's profile card, showing them where to find their smocks, and so on is time consuming. When you add the Welcome Packet to their visit, you can count on approximately ten minutes being taken up before the stylist actually comes to escort their new client to the service area. Adjustments on your appointment books need to be done in order to properly process all first-time clients. Your stylist must understand that, regardless of their schedule, the introductory period is equally important to the client's well-being. If the introduction is not done adequately, your salon risks losing clients, and income will be taken away from of other stylist who were not presented to the new client via the packet. Strong management is needed to prevent your staff from unwittingly defeating themselves by focusing on the moment, rather than on their entire careers.

Welcome Packets should be designed to expire, and the client must be made aware of this. Again, the purpose is to create multi-service clients. Without the expiration date, Welcome Packets can easily be tucked away and forgotten.

On the anniversary of your client's first service with your salon, send them a happy anniversary note with a "Circle of Friends" card tucked nicely inside.

You will also need to make a policy regarding whether they are transferable. Making them non-transferable protects you from giving discounts to visiting friends and relatives, while making them transferable encourages other family members to become part of your salon. It is your decision!

The Circle of Friends

On the anniversary of your client's first service with your salon, send them a happy anniversary note with a "Circle of Friends" card tucked nicely inside. By becoming part of this most welcomed group, they can receive benefits with your salon that others have yet to earn. As part of this program, you can recognize these individuals with beautiful extras that enhance each of their visits such as a complimentary hair conditioner with every service, 10% discount on all product purchases, seasonal gift packs, and even silent sales.

If you are computerized, knowing the anniversary date of each client is easy. You may decide to mail the cards to every person who has been part of your salon for one year, or you may choose to include only those with a certain number of visits to their credit, or a designated amount of money spent during the last twelve months. Clients who have reached the point where they are qualified to join your Circle of Friends have already demonstrated their loyalty to your salon. By offering them recognition and reward, you are deepening the bonds between you. Whether you adopt the program as it is suggested here or make up your own, the two most important elements that need to be included in your program are:

1. Systematically doing something extra for your loyal clients.
2. Doing it generously, although generous in this case does not imply "expensive." Products for your silent sales should be obtained through smart shopping and partnering with manufacturers. Your service costs can be offset by receiving special considerations for supplies.

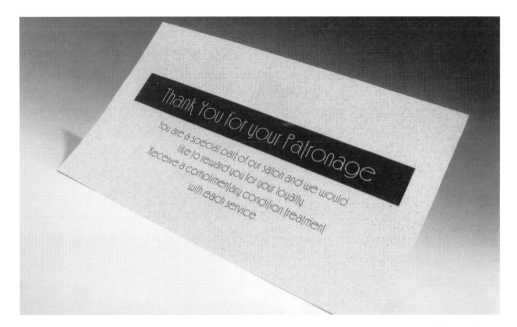

Thank you for your Patronage

You are a special part of our salon and we would like to reward you for your loyalty. Receive a complimentary condition treatment with each service.

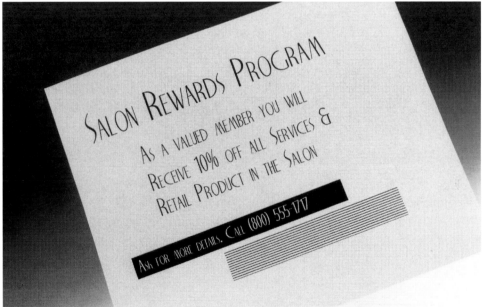

SALON REWARDS PROGRAM

As a valued member you will receive 10% off all Services & retail product in the Salon

Ask for more details. Call (800) 555-1717

Silent Sales

For all clients who belong to your Circle of Friends, it is especially nice to offer them the added benefit of silent sales. Like department stores, you can put key items on deal, without salon signs, and mail notices to all your loyal clients. It can be as simple as extending an extra 20% off (making it 30% total) on specified groups of products. Or, it could be a fantastic service offering such things as a complimentary body polishing with a paid body wrap service. Doing this once or twice a year, and making it well worth your clients' time, creates excitement, goodwill, and loyalty. By buying smart, you will be able to make a modest profit despite the generous discount, especially if you emphasize a brand name as part of your sale and approach your manufacturers for special pricing based on this marketing program.

SEASONAL GIFT PACKS

Seasonal gift packs are beautiful ways to say thank you to those who are part of your salon. They are also excellent tools for introducing new products, staff members, and services. Spring/Summer packs can be given out for a two-week period beginning March 15; Fall/Winter packs can begin September 15 (these dates, of course, are suggestions). Whatever dates you choose, a four-week span will help you reach half or more of your regular clients each year.

You may wish to give a seasonal gift to everyone who comes to your salon. But, a wiser course would be to establish a gift with purchase program such as those done in department stores. You could set a minimum purchase of $25.00, for instance, and then not only advertise your gift pack, but assign it a dollar value as well. For example: "Receive our spring gift pack, valued at $50.00, free when you purchase $25.00 or more in product before April 1." Seasonal gift packs also serve as wonderful incentives for clients to book appointments and try new services. Do not hesitate to send out mailers announcing their availability.

The Contents

A seasonal gift pack may contain gift slips toward services, a product gift (accompanied by a small coupon for their next purchase), or a free service appropriate to the season. All gift slips should have an expiration date of no more than forty-five days from the date of presentation. The packs may be put together in the same manner as other gift packs for your clients.

The seasonal pack works best when the gifts are selected carefully to enhance the theme your salon is promoting for a particular season.

Suggested seasonal pack contents for Spring/Summer include:

- ✦ Full-size thermal protectant spray.
- ✦ Travel-size collection of products.
- ✦ Sample packets of moisture-rich products.
- ✦ $10.00 gift slip towards a full highlighting service.
- ✦ $10.00 gift slip towards a body bronzing.
- ✦ $10.00 gift slip towards a body polishing.
- ✦ $10.00 gift slip towards a pedicure.
- ✦ Complimentary makeup application with new colors.

Suggested seasonal pack contents for Fall/Winter include:

- ✦ Full-size color-enhancing shampoo with $10.00 gift certificate towards color services.
- ✦ Styling aid good for fall hair fashions with a $10.00 gift certificate towards a translucent hair color treatment.
- ✦ $10.00 gift slip towards a facial.
- ✦ $5.00 gift slip towards a nail service.
- ✦ $10.00 gift slip towards a permanent wave.
- ✦ $10.00 gift slip towards a haircolor service.
- ✦ Therapeutic conditioning treatment.
- ✦ Complimentary makeup application with new colors with gift slip towards the purchase of makeup from the new collection.
- ✦ New Fall lipstick (compliments of your supplier) along with color chart and gift slip towards the purchase of makeup of their choice.

Strategies

While it is tempting to give everyone a seasonal gift pack twice a year and skip the Welcome Packet for all new clients, please resist. The Welcome Packet contains strategic gifts designed to introduce every new client to all aspects of your salon. After they have had that opportunity, the seasonal pack is there to thank them for their patronage. They are two different client care programs containing two distinct objectives. Make sure that you understand the difference, and that every staff member does, too.

All gift slips should have an expiration date of no more than forty-five days from the date of presentation.

EMBRACING THE PROGRAMS

Developing the expertise to negotiate cooperation and products from distributors and manufacturers takes time. Your salon must have a great record with most of these companies before complete benefits can be realized. For new companies that are eager for your business, validating your abilities can also elicit support. Putting your programs in writing, and making quality presentations will also count a long way in receiving their cooperation. Receiving written promises from your suppliers is equally important to the ongoing success of your gifting/promotional programs.

It takes manpower to run these programs and while your staff is still struggling with the basics, it is best to keep these exciting programs on hold until you are running smoothly in all other areas. Then, select one program at a time and implement it completely before adding another rewards program. Above all, allow your staff to enjoy the spirit of giving. Often, giving gifts is just as exciting as receiving them. Impart this spirit when you are explaining your

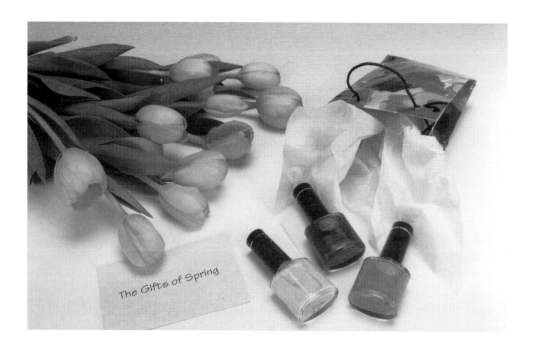

Figure 8-7
Spring seasonal pack gift.

The Gifts of Spring

newest gifting program and allow your staff to feel that they, too, are responsible for bringing these beautiful extras to their clientele.

chapter 9

Acts of Pleasure

1. Acts of wellness
2. Pleasing the five senses
3. Pleasurable details

HOTopic 4. Finishing touches

MORE THAN PAMPERING

Acts of pleasure include many things that address the needs of clients. They can mean comfort, gratification, and a heightened sense of well-being. Pleasure can be small acts, perhaps not even consciously perceived by your people, or they can be impressive parts of your menu, creating dramatic staying power for your clientele. Either way, acts of pleasure should pervade your salon and always be supported by your entire staff.

As discussed throughout this book, appealing to your clients' senses creates endless moments of pleasure for everyone. A clean smelling salon, gleaming chrome and mirrors, and a place that is orderly as well as attractive, are things that help clients enjoy their appointments. It is a draw that can distinguish your business from your competition. It is important to realize that great stylists can be found in every town, but a great business cannot.

ACTS OF WELLNESS

"Being alive" is a term coined by Faith Popcorn in her book *CLICKING*. She uses this phrase to describe society's trend of not only living longer, but wanting more quality of life while doing so. To fulfill part of this desire, people are seeking things that give them a sense of well-being. In our milieu, it can be de-stressing and detoxification services, plus numerous small details adding up to an entirely pleasurable and satisfying salon visit.

Aromatherapy Oils

Acts of well-being can be as simple as diffusing aromatherapy oils. Companies such as Aroma Vera and Aveda provide top-notch oils that can be purchased separately or blended to meet your needs. Electric diffusers are available from these companies and many others like them, to efficiently care for large areas in your salon. A timer can be obtained in any hardware store to ensure that the oils are intermittently diffused, creating a more subtle and pleasing fragrance.

Consider using natural aromatic sprays and abandoning the synthetic deodorizers you purchase at the grocery store.

Also consider using natural aromatic sprays in your restrooms and abandoning the synthetic deodorizers you purchase at the grocery store. Aromatherapy oils cost more than these cheaply produced items, but the difference is astounding once you become accustomed to natural blends. Your clients will recognize and appreciate the difference, too.

Creating a shampoo area that is far from the hubbub of the salon is also an excellent move. While you may not have the resources to create a separate room, you can create an independent environment. It begins with your stylists.

◆ Teach your staff how to prepare their clients for a nice, relaxing experience.

◆ Have them encourage clients to unwind and put the rest of their day aside.

◆ Train them to speak to clients in a relaxed, soft voice prior to the shampoo service to cue the client that this area of the salon is not a noisy, chatty place.

◆ Allow all clients to enjoy this experience every time they receive a hair service at your salon.

Just as successful salons and day spas such as Noelle Spa for Beauty and Wellness use aromatherapy candles in their shampoo areas, you should as well. The oils dispersed in this manner can promote balance, rejuvenation, or relaxation depending on the fragrances you choose. You can also include the technique shared by Adam Broderick Image Group of having each client inhale aromatherapy oils before the shampoo service actually begins (place drops of relaxing aromatherapy oils in the client's palms; then, ask them to cup their hands around their nose and take three deep breaths).

Therapeutic Massage

Also, allow your salon to smoothly transcend into a contemporary client care center by offering massage as part of your shampoo service. More than an act of pampering, massage is therapeutic. These manipulations can be used in conjunction with acupressure and can encourage lymphatic drainage. The massage portion of any shampoo service usually lasts only five minutes, but as we all know, it is often the most treasured part of the salon experience.

The important keys are to decide what type of massage you are going to do, it's benefits, and how long it will be performed. If you have a massage therapist, ask him to teach the staff several different types of massage for the head and neck (and the shoulders and arms). Consider organizing a half-day workshop, even if you have to hire someone from outside your business. Let your staff experience different massage techniques and ultimately create the ritual that will become a mainstay in your salon. Think in terms of quality, benefits, and time; make the service memorable yet practical.

Reducing Odors and Residue

Using low odor chemicals is a big plus in our business. Highly scented permanent waves are not suitable to the salon environment. Odor has nothing to do with effectiveness! If you find your staff requesting horrific smelling solutions, work with them in the selection of alternate, low odor products.

Establish firm policies with your nail department. Nail technicians often appear oblivious to acrylic odors, but the rest of the salon is not. If you feel acrylic nail services are necessary for your clientele, they must be controlled. This protects all people visiting and working in your environment from the strong fumes and acrylic dust this service generates.

Your responsibility is to adequately vent the nail area of your salon and to receive expert advice on how to do it. Research all advice carefully and ask for guarantees. The types of products nail technicians use are not always responsive to traditional venting methods.

One of the most ingenious methods of isolating nail odors comes from Salon India in Newport Beach, California. Their manicuring section is in a large alcove off the main waiting area. They simply put up a plexiglass wall with a doorway and vented the acrylic fumes directly to the outside of the building. Their nail care specialists are in full view of clients and no one is subjected to the by-products of their work. It is a perfect solution!

Hire nail technicians who only use low odor products. Make it clear that their products are not to be left uncovered, to evaporate into the air. Using simple devices such as product wells (small containers with caps that have a small hole at the top to insert the brush) are lifesavers when it comes to preserving the environment. However, never assume that this care will *always* be taken. Communicate, control, and follow up in this area at all times. By doing so, you will be protecting their business as well as your own.

The massage portion of any shampoo service usually lasts only five minutes, but it is often the most treasured part of the salon experience.

Lastly, nail technicians should never be placed openly next to the waiting area of your salon (unless you can isolate and vent their work area). This also holds true for anyone performing permanent wave services. These two odors are highly offensive to clients and should be done in areas set apart and specifically designed to have good air replacement capabilities.

Therapeutic Nail Services

Nail technicians can now offer a host of therapeutic add-on services, augmenting their clientele and improving services they already perform. There are mud masks for the hands and feet with enzymes to exfoliate, detoxify, and smooth skin. They can also offer aromatherapy manicures, and pedicures with leg wraps up to the knees, gel packs, and more to cool, soothe and beautify. Providing them with the best equipment will make their job more effective and profitable. The well-designed European pedicure chair is a great addition to your salon equipment. The comfort provided to the client is light years away from a simple salon chair and it allows your nail technicians to work with healthy postures.

Additionally, there are extended services, such as those offered at day spas. Nail technicians in these businesses often slough and moisturize the arms during manicures, adding value and benefit to their services. At Glen Ivy Hot Springs and Spa in Corona, California, nail technicians routinely exfoliate the skin up to the shoulders. When their trademark Glen Ivy Manicure is purchased, they also put aromatherapy oils in their finger bowl and perform a paraffin treatment along with a collagen mask on the hands. Their nail specialists also give a full 15-minute massage that has been therapeutically designed by their massage technicians. If you do the same, your pedicure and manicure business will soar. Providing your nail technicians with space that is relatively quiet will make it even better.

Therapeutic Hair Services

Hair services that embody wellness are also widely available. Companies such as Dermalogica offer products that detoxify the scalp and remineralize the skin and hair. There are numerous products that contain botanicals, and even more that include therapeutic substances high on their list of ingredients.

Offering therapeutic scalp treatments, such as the one given by the Oaks at Ojai Spa are also great ways to upgrade your service menu (the Oaks is a destination spa which also has a full-service hair salon). Their service lasts fifty minutes and is competitively priced with their chemical services. To heighten their service experience, they add a warm bubbling foot tub treated with aromatic sea salts. You can do this treatment, too. The only requirement is having a work area that is in harmony with the service.

Your responsibility is to adequately vent the nail area of your salon and to receive expert advice on how to do it.

Looking healthy is also important. Shine treatments for hair, such as those provided by the Shades EQ line by Redken, help people radiate a healthy appearance. Selling through to clients by sharing this benefit will aid enormously in increasing sales of this service in your salon. It is also often the finishing touch that makes the work your salon produces a cut above those of your competition. It is a detail in service you will not want to miss. Shine treatments are very profitable!

Use color products with conditioning agents and natural ingredients whenever possible; convey that you do through signage and your staff. Your menu of color services, along with the approach you take with them, will give you a competitive edge in the enormous color market that is absolutely here to stay. Adam Broderick Image Group has signage throughout it's salon that simply says, "Ask us about our Spa Color." They want their people to know that they perform haircoloring services that leave the hair and scalp in great condition. Their color business is booming. Yours can too!

There are also other things you can promote in your services as well as retail products. Makeup foundations that create healthy, natural color are extremely appealing, including bronzing powders, self-tanning products, and, of course, professional sunscreens. Educating your staff to apply makeup that radiates health is a natural service to accompany these sales.

Cross-Servicing

Cross-servicing pleasurable acts are also excellent ways to heighten the salon experience. GiGi Sims, esthetician for Toba Salon in Dana Point, California, frequently gives therapeutic hand massages to clients while their chemical services are processing. She also encourages all staff members to mist their clients' faces with a mixture of cool water and revitalizing essential oils after they have been under the dryer.

Noelle Spa for Beauty and Wellness offers every client, as part of their hair service, a paraffin hand dip performed with plastic gloves only. This treatment not only plumps up moisture in the skin, while providing great opportunities for bonding. Nail technicians can share their services via a hands-on introduction, as can estheticians.

Healthy Retail Stock

Servicing a contemporary clientele also means caring for their needs at home. Make sure that your retail products support a healthier lifestyle. Products with essential oils, herbs, minerals, and sea products will keep your retail business thriving. Body care products with therapeutic benefits also support this trend. Finishing products that have great ingredients, and promise glossy results, also

Use color products with conditioning agents and natural ingredients whenever possible; convey that you do through signage and your staff.

meet the needs of a contemporary clientele. The phrase "look and feel your best" has never been more appropriate.

Refreshments

Details of your shop can range from having aromatherapy teas and seasonal fruit to always serving fresh popcorn as people arrive for services in the early evening. Emotionally, this gesture of hospitality evokes warm, friendly feelings. On a more practical note, it takes the edge off early-evening hunger, making time spent in the salon more enjoyable.

Offering hot cider, fragrant teas, and coffee on cold blustery days are wonderful details that convey the message of sincere caring. Offering chilled beverages when weather is hot is also a pleasurable detail. Lemonade and iced tea are inexpensive to make, but the pleasure clients derive from drinking them on a warm summer's day is worth much more. Do not forget the value of chilled water. If you have ever been disappointed with a drinking fountain that only dispensed room temperature water, you will be more sensitive to this little act of pleasure. It is insignificant when compared to the excellent services you need to perform, but it is still part of the complex process that makes up extraordinary client care.

Reading Material

Reading material is also something that should be given careful thought. Not only does it need to consist of current issues, it should also be current with our times. More than likely, your salon services men and children. Do you have interesting, current reading material for them? Does your reading selection also include publications dealing with well-being? Do you offer a wide variety of fashion magazines? Do you refrain from putting professional beauty publications out for your clients to read?

FINISHING TOUCHES

Details can also include the many things already discussed in earlier chapters such as soft towels, attractive robes, and hand lotion in the restrooms. It can be something as simple as remaining safely protected during shampooing, or being offered fresh towels midway through chemical services. It can also mean skillfully managing the music in your salon to reflect not only the tastes of your clientele, but also the time of day.

To thriving businesses of the 21st century, details are the summation of their business style. Like personal relationships that are built on mutual experiences, client loyalty will reflect the care you have given to your business, right down to the very last detail.

Products with essential oils, herbs, minerals, and sea products will keep your retail business thriving.

The Art
of Retrieval

chapter 10

HOT*opic*

1. Creating a second chance for success
2. Method of retrieval
3. Enticements

SECOND CHANCES AT SUCCESS

Sometimes, despite our best efforts, we lose clientele. While some may leave because they are totally unhappy with their services, the majority of missing clients are far more likely to have dropped away because they simply were not satisfied enough to stay.

Retrieving these lost clients is an art that is easily mastered. It can be a highly effective program at your salon. In fact, return percentages of 70% or more are not uncommon with this practice. Retrievals also give you a second chance at winning over those you once disappointed and they present the opportunity of wisdom. Always make an effort to find out why these people have left your salon and remedy the situation!

When you first begin a retrieval program, brace yourself. Initially, you should include everyone who has failed to return to your salon even though their last visit may have been two years ago. If you are computerized, your job will be much easier to master. But, there will always be a great deal of auditing to be done by your front desk and artistic staff.

Eventually, your "missing" lists can be segregated by service, age, or gender, if you desire. In the beginning, run a general list of those clients who have not returned to your salon. And, if possible, run them by stylists.

- Do a few stylists have enormous lists while others have only a few missing?
- Check clients by service. Are there perm problems, color problems, or pre-booking problems?
- Do some lists have a lot of missing information? Are names misspelled? Were these clients neglected in other areas as well? Are they ghost entries?
- Have each stylist audit their own lists. Then have the front desk audit them. Do you have some clients who regularly come in at longer intervals? Are they simply not due for services? Be careful to double check names yourself that have been eliminated from the missing lists.

Once you established who is actually gone, take a moment to calculate your losses if you did not send incentives for them to return. For every 100 people and an average ticket price of only $40.00, your salon is missing $4,000 every six weeks. Multiply that by the entire year and the losses are overwhelming. Act smart and stop the losses before too much time elapses. Be generous in your thinking to make sure that those you once attracted will return to your business.

For every 100 people and an average ticket price of only $40.00, your salon is missing $4,000 every six weeks.

THE RETRIEVAL PROCESS

Once you have established your missing lists, categorize them by length of time gone. Prepare cards with a few different types of incentives, depending on how long the client has been absent from your salon (cards work best because they are cheaper to mail). Have information preprinted to speed up the preparation process.

The following section categorizes four different periods of missing time. For each mailing, you can use an identical card with three separate messages and colors. This often reduces the cost of the process and makes it easy to identify in your mailing bins. If you are computerized, have your mailing labels printed. To retain a personal touch, consider handwriting your messages and have them printed on your cards.

1. Missing six weeks

   When a client is gone for six weeks and does not have an appointment on the books, they should be contacted by telephone. Hopefully, you have established a formal waiting list. If so, running this client list is not necessary!

2. Missing eight to ten weeks

   Clients who are missing for eight to ten weeks need a little more prompting. By this time, if your system is in place, a reminder call has been made and still no appointment has been made. A simple card offering $5.00 off their next haircut appointment and a bottle of shampoo will bring many of them back. Expire the card in six weeks from the date of mailing. This is recommended because you may have already lost them for one haircut cycle, but you want to make sure they return to you during the next one. Always make this card non-transferable.

Salon Transcripts
Client Selection

Name/Last Visit	Address	City	Zip	Eve Phn	Day Phn
Adams, Kristen 4/26/97				555-1234	
Adams, Kristen 4/20/97	567 Main St.	Phoenix	99202		555-1234
Adams, Sally 4/26/97					
Allen, Leslie 4/24/97	567 Main St.	Phoenix	99202	555-1234	555-1234
Bartholomaus, Deanna 4/20/97	567 Main St.	Phoenix	99202	555-1234	
Becker, Lori 4/24/97	567 Main St.	Phoenix	99202	555-1234	
Becker, Mark 4/24/97	567 Main St.	Phoenix	99202	555-1234	555-1234
Berry, Mike 4/20/97	567 Main St.	Phoenix	99202	555-1234	
Beznaiguia, Cherie 4/26/97	567 Main St.	Phoenix	99202	555-1234	555-1234
Bold, Mike 4/21/97	567 Main St.	Phoenix	99202	555-1234	
Clark, Shawn 4/20/97	567 Main St.	Phoenix	99202	555-1234	
Clay, John 4/26/97	567 Main St.	Phoenix	99202	555-1234	
Clay, Mike 4/26/97	567 Main St.	Phoenix	99202	555-1234	
Friedland, Jessica 4/20/97	567 Main St.	Phoenix	99202	555-1234	555-1234
Golder, Debbie 4/20/97	567 Main St.	Phoenix	99202	555-1234	555-1234
Kelly, Ariana 4/20/97	567 Main St.	Phoenix	99202	555-1234	
Leonard, Stacy 4/21/97	567 Main St.	Phoenix	99202	555-1234	
Maxwell, Shawn 4/20/97	567 Main St.	Phoenix	99202	555-1234	555-1234
Paine, Paula 4/26/97	567 Main St.	Phoenix	99202	555-1234	
Pheles, Trish 4/26/97	567 Main St.	Phoenix	99202	555-1234	
Phelps, Tricia 4/21/97	567 Main St.	Phoenix	99202	555-1234	
Poole, Anna 4/20/97	567 Main St.	Phoenix	99202	555-1234	

22 clients selected or 2.51% of your clients.
Last Srvc Visit,emp:Jeff Mason between 4/20/97 and 4/27/97

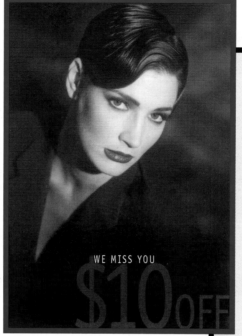

...and just to prove how

much we miss you,

_____

please redeem this card at your

next visit for $10.00 off on

your haircut *plus* a **gift** of an

8oz. bottle of shampoo!

Make your appointment

without delay!

offer expires: _____
non-transferable

WE MISS YOU

$10 OFF

Figure 10-1
A miss you card.

3. Missing twelve to sixteen weeks

Once gone this long, a greater incentive is needed to woo them back. Sending a card offering $10.00 towards their next hair service and a bottle of shampoo will bring even more missing clients back to your salon, especially when you include a sincere message with your gift. Do not forget to put an expiration date and make it non-transferable.

4. Missing twenty-four weeks (six months)

Keep a low profile but do not give up! At this point, the missing client can be treated as a shop client and not someone who is part of a particular stylist's clientele. For all stylists who are building, cards may be sent out on their be-half offering former clients a free haircut if they book with your new stylists. In reality, the haircut is only free if the client does not return. Remember the cost of attracting a new client! Giving a free service is still cheaper than purchasing advertisements.

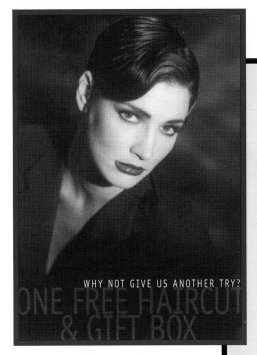

...and just to prove how

much we miss you,

_____

please redeem this card at your

next visit for $10.00 off on

your haircut *plus* a **gift** of an

8oz. bottle of shampoo!

Make your appointment

without delay!

offer expires: _____
non-transferable

Figure 10-2
Give us another try
card.

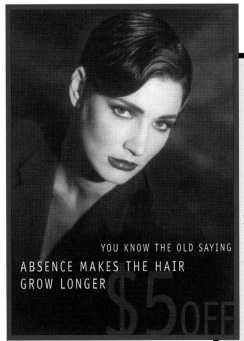

Our records indicate you're

overdue for services. Please make

your appointment today.

_____

Present this card during your next

appointment and receive

$5.00 off on

your haircut!

offer expires: _____
non-transferable

Figure 10-3
Overdue for services
card.

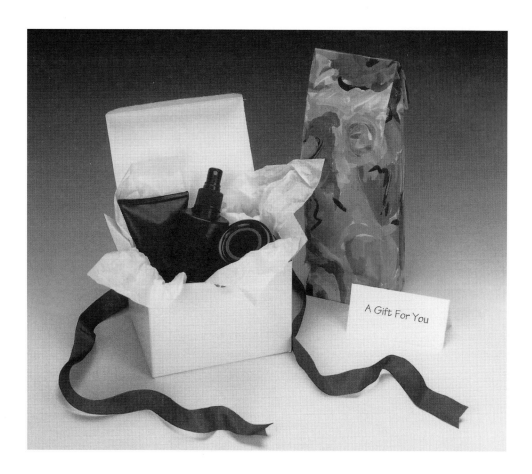

Figure 10-4
Client gift.

ACHIEVING RETENTION

By practicing your own contemporary client care program and following up on all the important details of your business, retrieving lost business will be easy and profitable. As your database stabilizes, your cash flow will continue to increase, especially if you continue to perfect and excel in your modern approach to client care.

Here is a timeline to help you use what you have learned.

Salon Timeline
Timeline : 0 to 6 months

☐ Delegate time. Revise your schedule to include several hours per week devoted only to doing the business side of your salon.

☐ Conduct a walk-through of your salon. Divide your salon into sections; then, test each area against your five senses.

☐ Check for timeliness of appointments.

- [ ] Establish a monthly routine of running complete computer reports. These should include:

    Client record cards

    Individual stylist client lists

    Percentage of services

    Retention rate of salon

    Retention rate of stylists

- [ ] Evalute Records. Check for completeness and accuracy.

- [ ] Devise ways to make your records more complete. Work with your front desk on booking and gathering information.

- [ ] Evalute your software. Does it provide you with all the information you need?

- [ ] Develop a client profile card.

- [ ] Evaluate yourself. Measure your commitment to running your business, to education, and the future of your business.

Timeline: 6 months to 1 year

- [ ] Create a schedule of excellence; including cleaning and maintenance of the salon.

- [ ] Establish guidelines of responsibility for cleanliness and maintenance for both the management and the staff.

- [ ] Establish guidelines for opening and closing your salon.

- [ ] Develop smart shopping habits. These should apply to purchasing salon supplies and salon goods.

- [ ] Scour your salon in search of "bits of waste."

- [ ] Develop and distribute client surveys.

- [ ] Establish and implement a program of client retrieval.

- [ ] Set salon goals.

- [ ] Make commitments to yourself, your staff, and your clients based on these goals.

- [ ] Develop your initial contemporary client care program. This includes adopting the "circle of care" and creating a broad-based plan.

- [ ] Create an educational program for staff members.

Timeline: 1 year to 18 months

- [ ] Continue to run and evaluate salon records. Check for accuracy and completeness and compare records from previous reports to measure growth.

☐ Have a meeting with your accountant once you are satisfied that your records are reasonably accurate. Discuss your profits and losses and evaluate percentages of expenses.

☐ Confer with your staff:

Establish a meeting plan.

Conduct a staff walk-through.

Work with staff to embrace the "circle of care."

Conduct step-by-step discussions.

Continue to create and distribute staff surveys in order to keep a close check on attitudes and ideas.

☐ Redefine the role of your front desk.

Define image.

Define responsibilities.

Continue to add details to the books.

Work towards smooth and timely check-ins and check-outs.

☐ Set up a regular meeting schedule for front desk personnel.

☐ Establish a system of client rewards.

☐ Create acts of wellness and pleasure for clients.

Timeline: 18 months and beyond

☐ Continue to revisit your contemporary client care plan. Make adjustments as necessary to keep it vital and effective.

Index

A

Advertising, 19

Anxiety, client, 7

Appointments, 43

Appreciation, acts of, 74

Aromatherapy oils, 126

Attitude, 43

B

Book checks, 44

Business

  cost of doing, 1-2

  evaluation, 9-15

By-products, 58-59, 61

C

Checklist

  client information, 43

  professional, 20000-21

  salon, 5-6, 11-14

  service supplies, 52

  shop supplies, 53

Checkout, 99-100

Chemicals, low odor, 127-28

Circle of care—a planned way to directly care for your clients and staff. 5, 21, 55-58, 80-93

Circle of Friends, 120-22

Cleanliness, 71-72, 80-83, 100-2

Client

  anxiety, 7

  appreciation, 65-66

  database, 34, 36-39

  information checklist, 43

  preparation for, 56-58

  profile card, 41-42

  questionnaire, 27-29

  record cards, 15-16

  rewarding, 50-51, 109-24

  retention, 18-19, 33-34, 36, 136-38

  surveys, 47-51

  welcoming, 59-63

Coding, 107

Communication, 64, 73, 87-89, 104-5

Computer

  capabilities, 25

  hardware components, 25

  software, 25-27

Computerization—automation. 23-40

Consultation—a vital discovery process that allows accurate information to be exchanged between stylist

and client. 64, 88-89

Contemporary client care—a program that consists of creating a beautiful environment that appeals to the

five senses. 5, 7, 55

Continuous care—taking your client at the appointed time. 62-63

Cross-servicing, 129

D

Database, 36-39. (See also Computer)

Dynamic draw, 2

E

Education, 65, 90-91

Efficiency tips, 58

F

Follow through, 69-70, 74, 91-93, 106-8

Front desk

  organization of training, 97-108

  redefining, 97

  team, 42-43

G

Ghost clients—clients who are incorrectly entered into the computer by way of improper spelling of a

name.

Gifts

gathering, 110-13

product, 113-14

seasonal, 122-23

Goals, salon, 70-71

Greetings, 61, 72

H

Hair services, therapeutic, 128-29

Hardware, computer, 25

History, salon, 2-4

Hospitality, 61-62

I

Image, defining, 98-99

M

Maintenance services, 45-47

Massage, therapeutic, 126-27

Meetings, establishing, 98

Morning greeter—a person in charge of preparing the salon before opening. 57

N

Nail, therapeutic services, 128

P

Packet, welcome, 117-20

Payroll, 19

Percentage of services, 18

Pleasurable acts, 63, 72-73, 86-87, 104

Prebooking, 66-69, 74, 91, 106

Product demonstration—a sales presentation. 112

Profit, 18-19

Program of care, defining, 76-77

Promotion, 19

R

Reading material, 130

Records, evaluating, 15

Referrals, 117

Refreshments, 130

Rent, 19

Responsibility, 46-47

Retail

  sales, 17

  stock, 129-30

  tickets, 29-31. (See also Service tickets)

Retention, 136-38. (See also Client, retention)

Retrieval, lost clients, 131-35

S

Salon

  analysis, 31-32

  checklist, 11-14, 17

cleanliness, 56-58

timing, 14-15

walk-through, 10

Service

excellence in, 73-74, 89-91, 105

maintenance, 45-47

supplies, 19, 51-52

tickets, 16-17, 29-31, 106

Shampoo area, 126

Software—programs recorded on diskettes, CDs, or the hard drive. 24-25 (See also Computer)

Staff

meetings, 77-79

scheduling, 57

Supplies

service, 19, 51-52

shop, 52-54

Surveys

client, 47-51

staff, 94-95

T

Team, front desk, 42-43

Therapeutic

hair service, 128-29

massage, 126-27

nail service, 128

Tickets, service, 16-17

Time

  coordinator, 44-45

  delegating, 24

  exercises in, 103

  running on, 72, 85-86, 103-4

Timing checklist, 14-15

Trade shows, 113

U

Utilities, 19

W

Waste, 53-54

Welcome, 59-63, 72, 83-85, 102. (See also Client, welcoming)

Welcome Packet, 117-20

Wellness, 63-64